Ketogenic Diet:

250+ Low-Carb, High-Fat Healthy Keto Recipes & Desserts + 100 Keto Tips, Tools, Resources & Mistakes to Avoid. (Ketogenic Cookbook, Lose Weight, Burn Fat, Ketosis, Ketogenic Recipes, Ketogenic Fat Bombs)

Kevin Hughes © 2016

All rights reserved. No part of this book may be reproduced in any form without permission in writing from the author. Reviewers may quote brief passages in reviews.

Disclaimer:

This book is for informational purposes only and the author, his agents, heirs, and assignees do not accept any responsibilities for any liabilities, actual or alleged, resulting from the use of this information.

This report is not "professional advice." The author encourages the reader to seek advice from a professional where any reasonably prudent person would do so. While every reasonable attempt has been made to verify the information contained in this eBook, the author and his affiliates cannot assume any responsibility for errors, inaccuracies or omissions, including omissions in transmission or reproduction.

Any references to people, events, organizations, or business entities are for educational and illustrative purposes only, and no intent to falsely characterize, recommend, disparage, or injure is intended or should be so construed. Any results stated or implied are consistent with general results, but this means results can and will vary. The author, his agents, and assigns, make no promises or guarantees, stated or implied. Individual results will vary and this work is supplied strictly on an "at your own risk" basis.

Introduction

First off, thanks for purchasing my book "Ketogenic Diet: 250+ Low-Carb, High-Fat Healthy Keto Recipes & Desserts + 100 Keto Tips, Tools, Resources & Mistakes to Avoid". By grabbing this book you've shown that you're serious about your diet and maintaining a healthy lifestyle. This book will teach you about the ketogenic diet and all of its benefits. I'll also be providing you with a ton of delicious recipes and other resources to help you get and stay on track. I hope this diet has the same positive impact on your life that it did on mine. I lost a ton of weight while also getting my blood sugar under control. Today, I have more energy and a fuller life because of what I learned while implementing this diet.

In this book, I will discuss the basics you need to know while also going over whether this particular diet is right for you. I'll be sharing 250+ recipes I've gathered over the years and a wealth of other resources you may find beneficial. I'll go over all the tools I use in my keto kitchen. I'll also be touching upon the pitfalls you'll want to avoid while starting out on this diet. I've included answers to many of the frequently asked questions I hear from those new to the ketogenic lifestyle.

It's important before beginning any diet you consult your physician. The ketogenic diet isn't suited for everyone. I'll go over this more in a later chapter but you should always ask your doctor if this diet is right for your specific set of circumstances. The goal is to get healthy. The last thing I'd want to see is someone following a diet that isn't helping them make positive progress towards that goal. I'm not a doctor, I'm just a person who's had success with the ketogenic diet. I've found that it allowed me to safely lose weight and get my other health issues under control.

If you're familiar with the ketogenic diet, I hope you enjoy all the recipes and resources I've included. They should keep you busy for the foreseeable future.

I'm excited to begin. Let's get started!

Chapter One: An Introduction to The Ketogenic Diet

What Is The Ketogenic Diet?

I often get asked what is the ketogenic diet? It's a high fat, low-carb diet that provides a variety of health benefits. During the last decade over 15 different studies have shown that this specific diet will not only allow you to lose weight but also improve your overall health. This diet is often used by people suffering from cancer, diabetes, Alzheimer's, and epilepsy.

The ketogenic diet also referred to as a keto diet, has similarities to both low-carb diets and the Atkins diet. This diet involves reducing the number of carbohydrates you take in and replacing those carbs with fat. Reducing your carbs in this fashion will place your body in a metabolic state known as ketosis.

So what is ketosis and why is it important? Ketosis happens when we have a low level of carbs in our system consistently. This causes us to deplete our liver glycogen leading to our body burning our fatty acids as fuel. This process creates ketones as the byproduct of that process. Ketones, like glucose, are a good source of fuel. A good way to look at ketosis is like flipping the switch in your body so that your only burning the fat in your body for fuel. When ketosis occurs our body becomes super efficient in burning our fat for more energy. This process also turns our fat into ketones in our liver, which can supply more energy to our brain.

The ketogenic diet can cause enormous reductions in both insulin and blood sugar levels. This, along with the increased amount of ketones, leads to several health benefits one can gain from sticking to this diet long term. Keto diets also lower cholesterol levels along with HDL and Triglyceride levels. Studies have shown that following this diet can be beneficial for people suffering from diabetes.

The ketogenic diet is an effective way to lose weight quickly and safely. It is superior to following a low-fat diet. Studies have shown that a keto diet is more filling than a normal diet so you're able to lose weight without having to keep track of calories. Those same studies have found that people following a keto diet lost more than 2 times the amount of weight than people following a reduced calorie low-fat diet.

The keto diet originated as a way of treating neurological diseases, like epilepsy. As years went by and the research on the diet grew, its been shown that following this diet could also help with other health issues. Here are a few of those conditions and why this diet is beneficial to those suffering from them. Remember to always check with your doctor before starting a new diet if you're suffering from one of these issues. Research is far from concrete and over time things get proved and disproved. While the research is positive it's in no way 100% conclusive.

Epilepsy - Studies show the keto diet can lead to a major reduction in seizures suffered by children with epilepsy.

Cancer - The keto diet is used when treating several forms of cancer to help slow the growth of tumors.

Heart disease - The keto diet can help improve many of the risk factors linked to heart disease. Among them, it can lower body fat, blood sugar, blood pressure, and HDL levels.

Alzheimer's - Studies show it helps to reduce the symptoms of patients suffering from Alzheimer's. It has been shown to slow down the progress of the disease.

Polycystic Ovary Syndrome - The keto diet can reduce our insulin levels. Insulin levels are thought to play a major role in this syndrome occurring.

Parkinson's - A few studies have shown a keto diet can improve the symptoms found in patients with Parkinson's.

Brain Injuries - There's been a recent study suggesting that a keto diet can aid in recovery from brain injury and help reduce the likelihood of a concussion.

Variations of the Ketogenic Diet

There is more than one ketogenic diet. In this section, I'll discuss a few of these variations and what they entail. This will help guide you to which version is best suited for your specific set of needs.

SKD or Standard Keto Diet - This version is low carb with moderate amounts of protein and high amounts of fat. It comprises 5% carbs, 20% protein, and 75% fat. This version is the one that has the most studies. It is the one I would recommend for most people wanting to try out the ketogenic diet for themselves.

High Protein Keto Diet - This version is like the standard keto diet but involves consuming a higher amount of protein. It comprises 5% carbs, 35% protein, and 60% fat.

CKD or Cyclical Keto Diet - This version involves having periods of higher carb days mixed in with your standard keto diet. For example, you would have 5 days of a standard keto diet followed by 2 days that are focused on consuming a higher amount of carbs. This version is favored by athletes and bodybuilders.

TKD or Targeted Keto Diet - This version lets you add in carbs around your workouts. This version is favored by athletes and bodybuilders.

Foods to Avoid

In this section, I will give you a list of foods you'll want to avoid while following the ketogenic diet. You'll want to avoid foods high in carbohydrates. The foods on this list should be avoided or had sparingly.

Fruit - Avoid all Fruits. Tiny portions of Strawberries or Berries is acceptable.

Starches & Grains - Rice, Wheat, Cereal, Pasta.

Root Vegetables - Sweet Potatoes, Potatoes, Parsnips, Carrots.

Legumes & Beans - Kidney Beans, Peas, Chickpeas, Lentils.

Sugar Filled Foods - Fruit Juice, Cake, Soda, Candy, Store Bought Ice Cream.

Unhealthy Fat - Processed Vegetable Oil and Mayonnaise.

Alcohol - These are often high in carbohydrates and can sometimes throw your body out of ketosis.

Diet or Items Labeled Low Fat - These items come highly processed and are normally loaded with carbs.

Sauces & Condiments - Avoid these as they often have unhealthy types of fat and sugar.

There are lots of food traps you must be careful of while on a ketogenic diet. Don't worry! I'll be giving you healthy alternatives. After a few weeks, you'll hardly notice these foods no longer being a part of your daily diet. Your body learns to readjust quickly. You'll be feeling so good you'll wonder why you didn't cut these foods out sooner.

Foods You Should Be Eating

In this section, I will go over a list of foods you should incorporate into your ketogenic diet. You'll want to stock up on these foods as many of them will become staples in your new diet. The foods on this list should become the base for the majority of all your future meals.

Meat - Red Meat, Ham, Steak, Sausage, Turkey, Chicken, and Bacon.

Fatty Fish - Trout, Salmon, Mackerel, and Tuna.

Eggs - Try to use omega-3 or pastured whole eggs.

Cream & Butter - Use grass fed.

Cheese - Goat, Cheddar, Cream, Mozzarella and Blue Cheese.

Seeds & Nuts - Walnuts, Almonds, Flaxseed, Chia Seeds, and Pumpkin Seeds.

Healthy Oils - Extra Virgin Olive Oil, Avocado Oil, and Coconut Oil.

Avocados - Fresh Guacamole or Whole Avocados.

Low-Carb Vegetables - Tomatoes, Green Vegetables, Peppers. and Onions.

Other - Spices, Herbs, Salt, and Pepper.

There's a lot of foods to choose from on this list. Creating interesting and delicious meals won't be an issue on the keto diet. In later chapters, I'll be giving you plenty of recipes to get you started. A great thing about this diet is that it leaves you feeling full. No longer do you need to associate going on a diet to starving.

Common Side Effects Of The Ketogenic Diet

Beginning a keto diet can be uncomfortable in the beginning. The reason is your metabolism is learning to burn fat instead of relying on using glucose. Most people often report feeling under the weather when first getting started. This phenomenon is known as "keto flu". It's your body going through withdrawals, much the same way someone addicted to drugs or alcohol would. Most people don't realize that their bodies are addicted to sugar and carbs. When you quit them abruptly your body reacts negatively. Your body also releases toxins as your fat cells are burned for energy.

That's why I suggest easing into your new ketogenic diet instead of going at it full steam. Introducing your body to a new diet slowly will allow your metabolism to handle the withdrawals without you having to suffer from the nasty side effects. Here are examples of what could happen when you start a ketogenic diet without easing into it. Remember, these side effects are only temporary. A byproduct of your body readjusting to your new dietary lifestyle.

Low Blood Sugar

Muscle Cramps

Dizziness

Diarrhea

Constipation

Frequent Urination

Sleep Issues

Fatigue

Headaches

Heart Palpitations

Shakiness

Sugar Cravings

Benefits Of The Ketogenic Diet

Once you've acclimated to your new diet, you'll notice all the wonderful benefits of living on a ketogenic diet. There have been many studies done over the years to back up that following this diet long term is beneficial to your overall health. In this section, I will list a few of the benefits you can achieve by following a ketogenic diet.

Weight Loss

Lack of Hunger

Increased Energy Levels

Lower Blood Pressure

Freedom From Food Cravings

Heartburn Relief

Increased Mental Clarity

Improved Sleep

Lower Cholesterol

Better Digestion

Better Dental Health

Less Stiffness and Joint Pain

Chapter Two: Getting Started On The Ketogenic Diet

The Basics to Getting Started

In this section, I'll be going over a couple things to consider before getting started along with the steps needed to make your transition as smooth as possible. There is a lot of different ways you can implement a keto diet into your life. A keto diet involves tracking the number of carbs in the food you eat and reducing your intake of these carbs to between 20 and 60 grams a day. Everyone is a little different so it may take a little experimentation to see how many carbs you can have each day and stay in ketosis.

The amount of protein you consume each day should be determined by what your goal is in terms of lean body mass or body weight. Your intake of protein will also differ depending on your gender, height, and activity level. Consuming too many grams of protein can also interfere with you remaining in ketosis. The balance of your calories after you calculate your protein and carb requirements will be from consuming fats. These ratios make sure that you not only go into a state of ketosis but you also stay in ketosis.

With a keto diet, the daily nutrient intake will usually work out to approximately 70% to 75% of your calories from fat, 20% to 25% of your calories from protein, and 5% to 10% of your calories from carbs. When on a keto diet you're not required to count your calories. You should, however, familiarize yourself by how your macronutrient percentages can become affected by your level of caloric intake. A low or high intake of calories will skewer your macronutrient percentages.

One key to implementing your keto diet plan correctly is to remember you're exchanging foods that contain carbs for a higher intake of fat and a moderate consumption of protein. So why moderate protein and high fat you ask? Well, fats have little to no effect on your insulin and blood sugar levels. Protein effects both so if you consume too much it will spike your levels and interfere with ketone production. If you eat too much protein without consuming enough fat you can make yourself sick and cause havoc on your metabolism.

I suggest getting a good carb counter. This will be a useful tool to have when you're first starting out. You want to get good at learning to count your carbs properly. I also suggest before beginning your diet you go through your kitchen and remove everything containing a high level of carbs. It will benefit you to restock your kitchen with the approved foods I listed in the last chapter. The fewer carbs in your home the better off you'll be.

The good thing about a ketogenic diet is that it doesn't require you to buy special kinds of foods. You don't need to waste your money on foods that come labeled as being low in carbs. There are a few exceptions like artificial sweeteners, but for the most part, a keto diet consists of less processed, natural food. The more natural foods you incorporate into your daily diet the healthier you'll be.

Being on a keto diet requires commitment. You'll be spending more time preparing your meals in your kitchen. Since you're eating natural foods, they won't already be processed and ready to go. I suggest brushing up on your cooking skills or taking a class if you have none. I love to cook so this one wasn't too big of a change for me. However, I have friends who had zero skills in the kitchen and they found this to be a daunting challenge at first.

I plan out my weekly meals on Friday nights. Each Saturday I shop for all my food and then I prepare the majority of my meals in advance on Sunday. Having a schedule and system in place makes the entire process go much smoother. It also ensures I always have a healthy meal on hand in case I'm feeling unmotivated to cook for myself at certain times of the week.

As with most diets, it's also very important to stay well hydrated when on this diet. The number of carbs you're consuming is lowered so your kidneys will naturally dump out the excess water it was retaining as the result of your previously high intake of carbs. I drink at least 8 glasses of water each day or 64 ounces. If you ever feel like you're getting a headache or a muscle cramp, it might be a sign you need to drink more water. You also might want to add more magnesium, salt, and potassium to your diet.

I also suggest keeping a daily log of your meals. I go over what I use in the resources section. Keeping track of what you're eating is a good tool to help keep you motivated and on point. It can also show you what types of things throw you off course. For instance, when I first started I noticed my caloric intake was terrible on Sunday. This was because for much of the year I would spend Sunday afternoons watching football with friends while eating and drinking non-stop. Once I saw what I was consuming compared to the rest of my week, I knew what changes I needed to make to keep me on track.

Don't forget to check with your physician before starting on this diet. I know it sounds like a giant hassle but you should always determine a proper course of action with a trained professional before getting started. My doctor recommended this diet as I had high blood pressure and high blood sugar levels. Now both issues are under control and I've lost a ton of extra weight. If I can do it so can you.

Chapter Three: 20 Ketogenic Diet Mistakes to Avoid

20 Ketogenic Diet Mistakes to Avoid

Learning to adjust to a keto lifestyle can be difficult at first. Like any other diet, there will be some things to learn and obstacles to overcome. Don't let disappointment or frustration derail you from your goal of a healthier lifestyle. In this section, I'm going to discuss many of the most common keto mistakes I see and what you can do to avoid them from dragging you down.

1. Obsessing About Your Weight - Your weight is one of the least effective ways to measure your progress. I only weigh myself once every two weeks. Doing it any more than that is essentially a waste of time as your weight will fluctuate with your water intake. Weighing yourself constantly will only lead to you feeling demoralized when the pounds aren't falling away as fast as you'd like them to. The safest way to lose weight long term is slowly over time.

2. Obsessing About Your Macros - You should always track your numbers. However, don't get obsessed over them. This is another psychological pitfall that will lead to you feeling depressed. Don't focus your mental energy on a preoccupation with food. Live your daily life and don't be shackled by what your current numbers are. Follow your diet and the results will come.

3. Not Increasing Your Fat Intake Slowly When Getting Started - Something I often hear about is people who run into an issue when first starting out on a keto diet. They often complain of bladder issues and having to go to the bathroom urgently. One solution to avoiding this situation is by slowly raising your daily fat intake over the course of two to three weeks. By allowing yourself to become "fat adapted" your body will become accustomed to breaking down the higher amounts of fat you're consuming in your new diet. This should stop you from having any unfortunate bathroom emergencies.

4. Consuming The Wrong Kinds of Fat - Eating fat isn't enough, you need to eat the proper kinds of fat. Steer clear of seed and vegetable oils. You want to stick to saturated fats. These are your animal fats, coconut oil, and butter. You also want to have plenty of monounsaturated fat. These are things like olive oil.

5. Not Eating Enough Fat - I know it's strange going from thinking how to avoid eating fat to trying to consume more of it as part of your keto diet. I had trouble with this at first. Just remind yourself that this is a diet that provides results and enjoy eating the extra fat. It may take a few weeks but you'll find those thoughts quickly fade away. Due to how our body responds to dietary fat, it's unlikely that you'll ever eat too much fat.

6. Only Focusing On Your Carb Intake - A keto diet relies on reducing the daily number of carbs you eat. However, a low-carb diet isn't enough to lose weight. Many people on zero-carb diets will end up gaining weight. A keto diet promotes a more moderate approach. Everyone is different so while no carbs may work for you, another person might need to add carbs to see the weight loss benefits. Most of the carbs in my diet come from non-starchy vegetables, seeds, berries, and nuts. These also have the benefit of being high in fiber.

7. Eating Too Much Protein - Protein is the most important macro you'll be consuming on this diet. It's essential for building and rebuilding our soft tissue (organs, muscles). Too much protein can sabotage your attempts at reaching ketosis. If you eat more protein than you need, any excess will get converted into glucose. For every 100 grams of protein, approximately 56 grams get converted to glucose. It's important to keep track and not overindulge.

8. Eating Foods That Are Processed - A keto diet is about eating real food. You should view it as eating ingredients. Try to avoid eating food that's processed. It's fine to occasionally have something processed but only if you have no better options available. I prepare all my meals on Sunday for the upcoming week. This way I know even if I'm feeling lazy or unmotivated during my week I don't have to worry about my meals because I've already prepared them. The more good habits you have in preparing your food the easier it'll be to stick to the diet.

9. Not Getting Enough Vitamins and Salt - People on a keto diet normally try to avoid salt, as too much salt in your body when inflamed can be bad for you. However, what most people fail to realize on this diet is that your body isn't inflamed, so you need more salt. You want to get at least 2 teaspoons each day. The same can be said for things like Vitamin D and magnesium. Make sure if you're not getting enough of these in your diet you're getting them through supplements.

10. Getting Worked Up Over Your Cholesterol - I hear this one quite a bit. Most people believe the myth that cholesterol is a horrible, dangerous thing. In fact, cholesterol is an essential part of what our body needs to survive. Having high cholesterol has no scientific correlation to cardiovascular or heart disease. The doctor who originally made this assertion rejected the same assertion once he realized there was no evidence to corroborate it.

11. Thinking A Keto Diet Is A Miracle Cure - A ketogenic diet is not a quick fix solution. This diet is a lifestyle change. This diet is not something to do to drop 10 pounds and then go back to your poor eating habits. The sooner you get serious about your long term health the better off you'll be.

12. Not Being Prepared For Ketosis - Some people often get the "keto flu" when first transitioning to this diet. While it can't always be avoided you can reduce the odds of having to go through it yourself. To do this you'll want to transition into your new ketogenic diet over the course of a few weeks. This will allow your body to avoid any withdrawals it may go through from cutting out carbs and sugar. It will also allow your body to acclimate to your new diet. I suggest drinking lots of water to help flush out toxins as they get released from the fat cells in your body. Doing these things should help you ward off most of the effects of the "keto flu". If you still have any issues you should also make sure you're getting enough sleep and monitor your salt intake for optimal levels.

13. Drinking Too Much - Alcohol is something to be avoided or had in moderation. Drinking too much will not only affect your ability to remain in ketosis but it also adds a lot of unnecessary sugars and carbs to your diet. Now I'm not saying you can't go out and enjoy yourself. However, try to keep your alcohol intake to a minimum.

14. Comparing Yourself With Other People - This is a dangerous trap that most of us have fallen prey to over and over again. It's difficult to not look at others and compare our progress with theirs. You need to stop doing it. Their success has no bearing on you and your success. Everyone is different and will progress slower or faster depending on their unique physical makeup. Just because you know someone else on a keto diet that's lost more weight than you in a shorter period time doesn't mean your results make you a failure. The sooner you get past this psychological roadblock the easier you'll be able to accomplish the goals you've set for yourself.

15. Not Giving 100% - This diet is not for those who aren't ready to commit to changing their lives. Going keto requires grit and determination. You are taking control of your life and health. To do so you need to be ready to make the hard choices and cut out a lot of the food you've spent the majority of your life eating. Not taking this diet seriously and not committing to staying on it can lead to you eating high-carb and high fat instead of eating low-carb and high fat. That would be a dangerous combination for your health.

16. Eating On A Schedule - Most of our lives we've been trained to eat three meals a day (breakfast, lunch, and dinner) with maybe a snack or two in-between. Well, I'm here to tell you that you don't need to live by those rules on a keto diet. If you're hungry eat. If you're not hungry, don't eat. It's as simple as that! Your body knows when you're hungry. Listen to it.

17. Doing It By Yourself - It's easier to make a big change like this if you have a support system in place. You need to reach out and find people going through the same struggles you are. It doesn't have to be a big support group, it only has to be big enough so you always have someone to help you stay motivated and on track when any difficulties arise. This can be a group of friends or family members. It can also be an online support group of people in a similar situation.

18. Allowing Setbacks to Impede Progress - Our success is often determined by how we handle our failures. If you were to give up on something every time you had a setback, there would be little that ever got accomplished. This piece of advice holds true when talking about diet. Being able to bounce back from failure is a vital component of any person's dieting success. None of us are perfect. There will be times when we fall off the wagon and stray from our diet. What matters is that we don't let our failure hold us back from dusting ourselves off and getting back to our diet.

19. Not Exercising - Having your diet under control is a wonderful accomplishment but to reap all the benefits of your lifestyle change you have to have an exercise regimen. Exercising will not only improve the effects of your dieting but it will give you greater mental clarity. The diet is the hard part. Find a physical activity you enjoy and do it regularly. I enjoy hiking so that's how I get a lot of my exercise each day.

20. Skipping The Intermittent Fast - This is one I hear about all the time. People try to skip out on fasting intermittently. I know it's not a fun thing to do but by fasting intermittently you're giving your body a much-needed break from digesting and breaking down all the food you consume on a daily basis. This is something I found to be very beneficial and I recommend trying it for yourself.

Chapter Four: Ketogenic Diet FAQ / Common Terms & Meanings

Ketogenic Diet FAQ

In this section, I will go over some of the common questions I come across the most when talking about the ketogenic diet. I hope you're able to find the answer to whatever remaining questions you have. If I missed something you should be able to find it on one of the sites or books, I recommend in the next chapter.

1. Will I Be Able to Eat Carbohydrates Again?

Yes, but it's important that you cut them out entirely when beginning this diet. A good time frame is about 2 to 3 months before you should have them again and then only on rare occasions. If you fall off the wagon, don't worry just pick yourself up and continue onward.

2. How Much Protein Am I Allowed to Eat?

You should only eat protein in moderation. Having a higher intake of protein can lead to lower ketones and a spike in your insulin levels. About 35% of your total caloric intake is about the upper limit.

3. Do I need to Carb Load or Refeed On This Diet?

No. However, having a few days that are higher calorie can be beneficial to you every once in a while.

4. Will This Diet Cause Me to Lose Muscle?

Every diet comes with the risk of losing at least some of your muscle. Since this diet focuses on eating high levels of protein it may aid in minimizing your muscle loss. If you're that concerned, try lifting weights as one of your forms of exercise.

5. Am I Able to Build Muscle On A Keto Diet?

Yes, however, it can be harder to do than if you were on a diet with a moderate amount of carbs.

6. I Thought Ketosis Was Dangerous. Is That True?

Many people get ketosis confused with ketoacidosis. Ketosis is a natural and perfectly healthy when on this diet. The latter will only occur in people with a case of diabetes that has gone uncontrolled. Ketoacidosis can be very dangerous.

7. What If I Constantly Feel Weak, Fatigued, or Tired?

If you feel this way, your body may not fully in ketosis and using your ketones and fats efficiently. To combat this, try lowering your intake of carbs. You may also want to try using an MCT oil supplement for additional help. Another good suggestion is to eat salty items and stay hydrated. This will help combat some of the side effects you're feeling.

8. My Breath Smells. Is There Anything I Can Do?

This reaction is a normal side effect. Chew sugar-free gum or drink water that is naturally flavored.

9. My Urine Has A Fruity Smell? Is This Normal?

Yes, this is normal. It is due to you excreting the byproducts that are created while in ketosis.

10. I Have Diarrhea and Digestion Problems. Can I Do Something?

This is a normal side effect. It will subside in 3 to 4 weeks. If it continues on past this you should eat more vegetables high in fiber. You may also want to consider a magnesium supplement if you find yourself constipated.

11. How Long Does Ketosis Take to Occur?

A keto diet isn't something you can start and stop at a whim. Your body needs time to adjust if you want to reach the metabolic state of ketosis. This process may take between 2 and 7 days. It all depends on your activity level, body type, and foods you're eating. The quickest way into ketosis is by exercising while on an empty stomach. You'll also want to restrict your intake of carbs to less than 20g a day while drinking plenty of water.

12. How Do I Keep Track Of My Carbohydrates?

I use a free app called MyFitnessPal. It's both web-based and mobile so I can track everything no matter what I'm doing. To track your net amount of carbs, subtract your total intake of fiber for the day from your total intake of carbs for the day. I'm sure there's plenty of other apps and trackers you can use to do the same thing but this is the one I have experience with. Look around and see if you find one more suited to you.

13. Will I Need to Always Count My Calories?

No matter what diet you're on calories matter. That being said, with a keto diet you rarely must worry about your calorie intake because the proteins and fats you consume will keep you feeling full for long periods of time. If you exercise frequently remember that you're burning calories so you must make sure you're eating enough to make up for this deficit.

14. How Much Weight Can I Expect to Lose?

The answer to this is dependent on you. Weight loss will fluctuate depending on your level of exercise and your specific metabolism. One tip to help you out is try cutting out things that cause your weight loss to stall. These things are wheat products, dairy, and artificial sweeteners.

15. Is It Possible to Eat Too Much Fat?

Yes. When you eat too much fat, it will push you from being in a calorie deficit to a surplus. Most people find it's hard to overeat on a Keto diet but it's possible. If you're worried about that you can always use your keto calculator to figure out how many proteins, fats, and carbohydrates you need to eat each day. I'll be sharing a keto calculator in the next chapter's resource section.

16. What Should I Do If I Stop Losing Weight?

This is a common issue. In every diet, weight loss will slow or stop from time to time. If you find you're struggling to lose weight I suggest changing up your methods. Try cutting certain foods out of your diet to see if it helps. Another effective tip is to change up your eating patterns. These setbacks are only temporary roadblocks. Don't get too stressed out if you plateau from time to time.

Here are ideas on what to do if you stop losing weight.

Remove Dairy From Your Diet

Up Your Intake Of Fat

Decrease Your Intake Of Carbs

Cut Out Gluten

Stop Eating Any Nuts

Look For Any Hidden Carbs

Cut Processed Food Out Of Your Diet

Cut Out Any Artificial Sweeteners

Measuring Food Instead of Weighing It.

17. How Can I Tell if I Am In Ketosis?

I like to use a Ketostix. These can be found online or at your pharmacy. These are not very accurate but they'll give you a good idea if you're in ketosis. For a more accurate reading, you can get a blood ketone meter. I'll go over what I use in the next chapter.

If you get a blood ketone meter, here is what all the readings will mean:

Light Ketosis - .5 mmol/L to .8 mmol/L - Not ideal for weight loss.

Medium Ketosis - .9 mmol/L to 1.4 mmol/L - This is fine for weight loss.

Deep Ketosis - 1.5 mmol/L to 3 mmol/L - This is the ideal state for weight loss.

18. Am I At Risk For Heart Issues From Eating So Much Fat?

Fat is broken up into 3 main different groups. These are monounsaturated fats, polyunsaturated fats, and saturated fats. Let's go over each of the three.

Saturated Fats - Recent studies show these improve your cholesterol and don't lead to heart attacks. Eat these without worry.

Monounsaturated Fats - Considered healthy fats. Can help to lower cholesterol. Olive oil is one example of these.

Polyunsaturated Fats - When processed these are bad for us. This includes vegetable oils and margarine spreads. When processed they are linked to heart issues and therefore should be avoided. The same goes for trans fats. On the flip side when polyunsaturated fats occur in nature they are shown to improve cholesterol. These include foods such as fish.

19. What The Heck Are Macros and Should I Be Counting Them?

Macros is short for macronutrients. The 3 main macros are carbs, proteins, and fats. It's best when first starting out you track all three macros along with your calories. Doing so will help you form healthier eating habits and give you a better idea of how you're sticking to the diet. It's easy to lie to ourselves and forget things if we don't keep track.

Another reason to track our macros is to help us figure out how to proceed when our weight plateaus. The more data on hand, the better you'll be able to decide on how to adjust your diet. When tracking macros, think in terms of grams and not percentages. Grams will give you the best idea of everything you're eating.

Don't get too obsessed with your macros. You have room. If you're a little over or under one day, don't get bent out of shape. As long as you're also keeping count of your calories you won't fall into a deficit and you'll be just fine.

20. Am I Allowed to Drink Alcohol On A Keto Diet?

Yes, you can consume alcohol but be careful. Alcohol contains hidden carbs. If you are drinking alcohol, it's best to stick with clear liquor. Try to stay away from flavored liquor, wine, cocktails, and beer as these all contain carbs.

21. I Exercise Regularly, Do I Need to Be Worried?

People who exercise fall into two main categories. Those who focus on cardio and those who focusing on weight lifting. If you fall into the cardio category you have nothing to worry about. Studies have shown that people who do aerobic training aren't affected by going on a low-carb diet.

Now if you lift weights, you need to know what your goal is. Carbs will allow you to recover faster and make faster gains so there's benefit to trying one of these two variations on the ketogenic diet. One is a Cyclical Keto Diet, the other is a Targeted Keto Diet.

TKD is when you're having just enough carbs prior to your workout to get you out of ketosis for your workout's duration. This works by supplying a glycogen source for your muscles to use and once it is used up, you'll go back into ketosis. This is the method I would suggest to people who lift as part of their normal exercise routine but aren't trying to become ripped bodybuilders.

CKD is a more advanced. I suggest only people experienced with the keto diet try using this method. It's aimed more at competitive bodybuilders than normal people. In this method, you follow your normal keto diet for 5 days and then switch to a carb heavy diet for the other 2 days. You're replenishing all the glycogen stores in your body for the training you'll do during the rest of your week.

22. What Types Of Supplements Should I Be Taking?

People on a keto diet will often go through a period of readjustment where they feel off. If you're cramping or feeling not quite like yourself here are some supplements, you can try adding to your regiment. Before starting any new supplements you should always consult your doctor or physician.

Multivitamin

Vitamin D Supplement

Vitamin B Complex

Magnesium Supplement

Potassium Supplement

Common Terms & Meanings

AS - Stands for Artificial Sweetener. These are used to help sweeten food and reduce or eliminate our use of carbs.

BPC - Stands for Bulletproof Coffee. This is oil, coffee, and butter mixed using an emulsion blender to raise your fat content. This is done to make you feel "full" in the morning so you don't have the urge to overeat.

Fat Bomb - These are full of fats and oil to raise our daily fat content. People who have trouble having enough fat use these to help themselves out. These need not be sweet. Make them to your preference. I prefer mine a little salty.

HWC - This means Heavy Whipping Cream. This is a staple as I use cream in my coffee every day.

IR - Stands for Insulin Resistance. This is when our body's cells aren't able to respond to insulin hormone.

LCHF - Stands for Low-Carb High-Fat. The whole concept of what a keto diet is.

MCT - Stands for Medium Chain Triglyceride. Helps boost our metabolism. Once metabolized they turn into ketones.

SF - Stands for Sugar-Free. Tons of options for sugar-free foods available.

WOE - Stands for Way of Eating. A term that is used to help reference our personal diet.

Chapter Five: A Guide to Ketogenic Diet Tools, Resources, Apps, & Books

Ketogenic Diet Kitchen Tools Guide

In this section, I will go over some of the kitchen tools I use regularly. You'll find many of these referenced at certain times in the recipes I will share with you. I gained these over time so grab the one's most important to you and add new items as you get the chance. Having these items will increase the number of recipes you can make while making the entire process simpler and faster. I've shared the models I use along with links to them and their current pricing. Over time, some of these prices might fluctuate and newer more efficient models may be released. Always do your research and determine what brands and models best suit your specific set of needs. This is not a complete list. I'm sure I forgot about something or don't own it in my kitchen.

Bacon Press - Bacon is one of my favorite foods so this is a necessity in my household. I use a Norpro Cast Iron Round Bacon Grill Press. Costs about $15.00.

Bakeware Set- A must have. I use a KitchenAid KB6NSS5 Classic Nonstick 5-piece Bakeware Set. Costs about $60.00.

Casserole Dish - I use this at least once a week. I have a Pyrex Bakeware 4.8 Quart Oblong Casserole Dish. Costs about $10.00.

Cast Iron Pan - Another necessary tool to own in your keto kitchen. I use a 12 inch Calphalon Pre-Seasoned Cast Iron Cookware Skillet. Costs about $30.00.

Cheese Knives - A good tool to have. I use a set of 4 Prodyne K-4-S Stainless Steel Cheese Knives. Costs about $13.00.

Cheese Slicer -A great recent addition to my kitchen. I use a Bellemain Adjustable Thickness Cheese Slicer. Costs about $9.00.

Coffee Maker - I can't remember my life before coffee. I use a Keurig K60/K65 Special Edition & Signature Brewers Single-Cup Brewing System. Costs around $330.00. I use a high-end model, you can find many excellent cheaper versions.

Containers - A must have in any kitchen. I use Kinetic GoGREEN Glassworks Series Oven Safe Glass Food Storage Container Set 15-Ounce Each (3 Containers and 3 Lids). Costs about $$24.00. I have a few sets of these along with my Rubbermaid containers.

Convection Oven - A wonderful addition to my keto kitchen. I use a Black & Decker CTO6335S Stainless Steel Countertop Convection Oven. Costs about $80.00.

Crockpot - I love using my crockpot. One of the first items I purchased for my kitchen. I use a Crock-Pot SCV700SS 7-Quart Oval Manual Slow Cooker. Costs about $50.00.

Cutting Board - A must have. I use an Epicurean 12 by 9-Inch NonSlip Gripper Cutting Board. Costs about $25.00.

Food Processor - I use a Cuisinart DLC-10S Pro Classic 7-Cup Food Processor. I find it comes in handy with a lot of the recipes I make and cuts down on my prep time. Costs about $170.00.

Food Scale - Something I use daily. I have an Ozeri Pronto Digital Multifunction Kitchen and Food Scale. Costs about $12.00.

Food Storage Set - A great item to keep your food stored. I use a 42 piece Rubbermaid Easy Find Lid Food Storage Container Set. Costs about $16.00.

Food Thermometer - A must have. I use a Lavatools Javelin Digital Instant Read Food and Meat Thermometer. Costs about $25.00.

Fryer - Having a fryer allows you to create so many new and interesting dishes. I use a Hamilton Beach 35034 Professional-Style Deep Fryer. Costs about $55.00.

Grease Keeper - Great addition to my kitchen. I use an RSVP Stoneware Grease Keeper. Costs about $22.00.

Immersion Blender - Great tool to have in your arsenal. I find I use it often. I have a Kitchen Aid KHB2351CU 3-Speed Hand Blender. Costs about $60.00.

Indoor Grill - Having an indoor version comes in handy during those cold winter months. I use a Hamilton Beach 25360 Indoor Flavor Searing Grill. Costs about $62.00.

Knife Set - This is a must. You're only as good as your tools. I use a VonShef 9 Piece Professional Kitchen Knife Carry Set. Costs about $240.00. I got this as a gift. I'm sure there are wonderful knife sets you can find on a smaller budget.

Knife Sharpener - If you're going to spend good money on a set of knives you need to keep them sharp. I use a Harcas Knife Sharpener Professional 2 Stage Sharpening System. Costs about $13.00.

Magic Bullet Nutribullet - I use this one at least once a week. I have a Magic Bullet Nutribullet 12-Piece High-Speed Blender Mixer System. Costs about $80.00.

Mandoline - Comes in handy. I use an OXO Good Grips V-Blade Mandoline Slicer. Costs about $40.00.

Measuring Cups - Another must own kitchen tool. I use a Kitchen Made 7 Piece Stainless Steel-Nesting Set. Costs about $28.00.

Measuring Spoons - Another must own kitchen tool. I use the Utopia Kitchen Professional Grade Stainless Steel 6-Piece Measuring Spoon Set. Costs about $8.00.

Metal Skewers - I love making kabobs so I use mine all the time. I have UPI Long Shish Kebab Kabob Skewers. Costs about $7.00 per dozen.

Mixing Bowl Set - This is a must have. I use a set of ChefLand Mixing Bowls. Costs about $20.00.

Muffin Pans - A must have. Invest in some good muffin pans, you'll be happy you did. I use a 12 Cup USA Pan Bakeware Aluminized Steel Cupcake and Muffin Pan. Costs around $23.00.

Potato Masher - Nice tool. I use an Orblue Potato Masher. Costs about $12.00.

Ramekins - I use these often. I have two sets of 6 Bellemain 4 oz. Porcelain Ramekins. Each set costs about $13.00.

Roaster Pan - Great recent addition to my kitchen. I use a Calphalon Classic Hard Anodized 16-Inch Roaster with Nonstick Rack. Costs about 60.00.

Silicone Baking Cups - Wonderful addition to my kitchen. I use Pantry Elements Silicone Baking Cups / Cupcake Liners. Costs about $8.00.

Silicone Egg Ring - Perfect for making round perfect eggs. I use a Joie Roundy Silicone Egg Ring. Costs about $6.00.

Silicone Spatula - Love these. I use a Chef Series Flex Turner Spatulas 3 Piece Set. Costs about $30.00.

Spiralizer - Another amazing tool. I don't use it often but it comes in handy when I need it. I use this to make my zoodles. I use a WonderVeg Vegetable Spiralizer. Costs about $24.00.

Stockpot - I use this all time. I have a 8 quart Specialty Total Nonstick Dishwasher Safe Oven Safe Stockpot Cookware. Costs about $30.00.

Timer - An excellent tool. I use a ThermoWorks TimeStick. Costs about $55.00. There's plenty of cheaper alternatives out there.

Twine - I don't need this often but it's nice to have on hand when I do. I use Norpro Stainless-Steel Holder with Cotton Cooking Twine, 220 feet. Costs about $12.00.

Vidalia Chop Wizard - Love this tool. Makes chopping go much faster. Costs about $20.00.

Vitamix - A must have in my kitchen. I often use mine to make homemade ice cream, soups, and whole-food juices. Has a lot of great features. I use a Vitamix Professional Series 750. Costs about $600.00.

Waffle Maker - Some great recipes out there for ketogenic approved waffles. I use a Presto 03510 FlipSide Belgian Waffle Maker. Costs about $52.00.

Whip Cream Maker - Great tool for desserts. I use iSi Mini Easy Whip, 1/2-Pint Cream Whipper. Costs about $40.00

Zoku Pop Maker - Fast ice pop maker. I use this in a few of my recipes. Was an excellent addition to my kitchen. Costs around $35 and will allow you to make healthy pops in under 10 minutes.

Ketogenic Diet Testing Tools & Supplements Guide

Blood Ketone Meter - A good tool to have in your arsenal. I use Precision Xtra Blood Glucose and Ketone Monitoring System. Costs about $26.00.

KetoStix - An easy way to test if you're in ketosis. I use Ketostix Reagent Strips. Costs about $20.00 and comes with 100 strips.

MCT Oil - I've used this a bunch over the years. I use Premium Organic MCT Oil. Costs about $25.00.

Multivitamin - I like to take a multivitamin targeted for people on a keto diet. I use Ketolabs Keto Core Daily Multivitamin. Costs about $50.00.

Ketogenic Diet Resource Guide

In this section, I will go over my favorites sites and resources related to the ketogenic diet. There's a wealth of information on the subject. If you have a question, I'd be surprised if you couldn't find it using one of these resources.

Keto Diet Resource - An excellent site, loaded with a ton of information. Helped me out when I first got started. You can find it here: http://www.ketogenic-diet-resource.com/

Caveman Keto - A great site I frequent regularly. Filled with tons of resources to help you out along the way. A definite must in my book. You can find it here: http://cavemanketo.com/

Ruled.me - A wonderful site dedicated to the ketogenic diet. Filled with recipes, articles, and guides on how to go about following a keto diet. You can find it here: http://www.ruled.me/

Keto Calculator - Awesome keto calculator. Easy to use and understand. You can find it here: http://www.ruled.me/keto-calculator/

Ketogenic Diet Facebook Group - Great place to share your stories and recipes. Very motivating. You can find it here: https://www.facebook.com/Ketogenic-diet-Low-Carb-Living-649623888417983/

Ketogenic Diet App Guide

In this section, I'm going to discuss my favorite apps related to the ketogenic diet. These are apps that I've tried out myself at one point. I'm sure there are others I may have missed but this guide will give you a good idea of the different apps available to you. I suggest trying a few and sticking with those that best suit your needs.

MyFitnessPal - This is a free app and my favorite of the bunch. It can track your food, exercise, measurements, and weight. A great calorie counter that can be changed to track you on your keto diet. Available as both a web-based app and on your iOS and Android mobile devices. Here's a link to an article on how to change it for your keto needs.

Carb Manager - Excellent for tracking your carbs and staying on top of your keto diet. On iPad and iOS for $2.99. Also comes with in-app purchases.

Keto Diet App - Full version available on iPad only for $4.99. It's supposed to be coming to the iOS and Android in the near future. The basic version is available on both iOS and Android for $1.99. Both options offer a ton of helpful features and resources to make following your diet easier.

Ketogenic Diet Recipes App - Over 200 delicious ketogenic diet recipes at your fingertips. Only for the iOS. Costs $1.99.

Ketogenic Diet Calculator - A simple to use calculator when you're on the move and need to figure out the keto ratios for your meal. Only for the iOS. Costs $1.99.

Stupid Simple Keto - On both iOS and Android. This is a free app with in-app purchases. This app makes tracking your food easy and offers a bevy of features.

MyPlate Calorie Counter - A free web-based app that allows you to track not only your calories but your cholesterol, sugar, and calcium. Comes with nutritional charts and other helpful information.

Ketogenic Diet Book Guide

Here are a few of my favorite books on the keto diet. I've read a lot on this subject over the years and these are a few of the books that made an impression. I hope they do the same for you.

The Protein Power Lifeplan by Dr. Michael and Mary Dan Eades

The Art and Science of Low Carbohydrate Living: An Expert Guide to Making the Life-Saving Benefits of Carbohydrate Restriction Sustainable and Enjoyable by Dr. Jeff Volek and Dr. Stephen Phinney

Dr. Atkins' New Diet Revolution, Revised Edition by Dr. Robert Atkins

Chapter Six: Ketogenic Diet Breakfast Recipes

In this section, I will give you 50 ketogenic breakfast recipes you can make yourself. I'll include both basic recipes and a few more advanced recipes. That way no matter what your level in the kitchen you'll be able to prepare healthy low carb keto meals to keep you on track with your diet. I'll add in the nutritional value whenever possible, although I don't have those exact numbers for every recipe.

Delightful Scrambled Eggs

Ingredients:

3 large Eggs

Fresh Ground Pepper

Coarse Salt

1 tablespoon of Unsalted Butter

Directions:

1. Beat eggs using a fork.

2. Melt your butter using a nonstick medium skillet on low heat.

3. Add in your egg mixture.

4. Using your spatula (preferably flexible and heatproof), gently move eggs into center of your pan and allow the liquid parts to run out to the perimeter. Continue to cook moving your eggs with your spatula until they are set. Should take approximately 1 1/2 minutes to 3 minutes.

5. Season your eggs with pepper and salt.

6. Serve and Enjoy!

Nutritional Value:

17.5 grams of Protein.

26.3 grams of Fat.

1.8 grams of Carbs.

318 Calories.

Spinach Egg White Omelet

Ingredients:

4 - 5 Egg Whites

1 Egg Yolk

1/2 Tomato or 1 Plum Tomato

2 tablespoons of Almond Milk - Can substitute with Coconut Milk, Skim Milk, or Soy Milk

1 handful of Shredded Spinach

1 pinch of Basil

1 tablespoon of Purple Onion

Olive Oil Cook Spray

Garlic (optional)

Directions:

1. Chop up your vegetables.

2. Beat your egg whites, yolk. and almond milk.

3. Spray your small sized frying pan with olive oil spray and saute your vegetables until they get soft.

4. Put your vegetables to the side.

5. Spray your pan again with olive oil spray.

6. Place heat on medium-low and pour in your eggs mixture. Cook the eggs until firm, then add your vegetables on one side of eggs and fold the other side of the eggs over top.

7. Add to your plate.

8. Serve and Enjoy!

Nutritional Value:

20 grams of Protein.

5 grams of Fat.

18 grams of Carbs.

203 Calories.

Egg Muffin Cups - (Makes 6)

Ingredients:

6 Eggs

1/2 cup of Sliced Spinach

6 slices of Shaved Nitrate Free Turkey

Light Mozzarella Cheese

2 tablespoons of Red Onion

3 tablespoons of Red Pepper

Fresh Pepper

Salt

Olive Oil Spray

Fresh Basil (optional)

Directions:

1. Preheat your oven to 350 degrees.

2. Slice your spinach, grate your mozzarella cheese and prepare your red onion and red pepper.

3. Get a nonstick muffin tin and spray with olive oil.

4. Place turkey in one of the muffin tin cups. Make sure it's resting both on the sides and bottom of your tin.

5. Crack 1 egg and pour into your newly made turkey cup. Repeat this with each egg into it's own cup.

6. Add some spinach, red pepper, cheese, and red onion on top of each egg.

7. Season each egg with salt and fresh pepper. Can also add basil if you're using it.

8. Place your tin into the oven and continue to bake till your eggs are all set and their whites are an opaque color. Should be about 10 minutes to get a runnier yolk and around 15 minutes if you want a harder yolk. Be aware that each egg muffin will continue cooking for a short time after they've left the oven.

9. Serve and Enjoy!

Nutritional Value: (1 Egg Muffin Cup).

9 grams of Protein.

6 grams of Fat.

2 grams of Carbs.

95 Calories.

Perfected Scrambled Eggs (Serves 2)

Ingredients:

6 Eggs

2 tablespoons of Sour Cream

2 tablespoons of Butter

1/2 teaspoon of Salt

4 strips of Bacon

1/2 teaspoon of Onion Powder

1/2 teaspoon of Garlic Powder

1/4 teaspoon of Black Pepper

1/4 teaspoon of Paprika

Directions:

1. Crack your eggs in an ungreased, cold pan and then add your butter. Wait to mix eggs till you put the heat on. Don't season the eggs until after cooked it will break them down and make them watery instead of creamy.

2. Put your pan on medium-high heat. Start stirring the butter and eggs together using preferably a silicone spatula. While stirring your eggs, cook some bacon strips in a different pan to your desired level of crispiness.

3. Alternate stirring your eggs both on heat and off the heat. A few seconds on and a few seconds off the flame. If the eggs begin cooking in a thin, dry looking layer at the bottom of your pan, take if off heat. Scrape it using your spatula and that thin layer should regain some of its creaminess.

4. Once the eggs are almost done turn off the flame. Your eggs will cook a little more due to residual heat in your pan.

5. Add 2 tablespoons of your sour cream. Season your eggs using the pepper, salt, paprika, onion powder, and garlic powder.

6. You can add in a couple stalks of chopped green onion for some contrasting flavor.

7. Serve and Enjoy!

Nutritional Value:

25 grams of Protein.

35 grams of Fat.

2 grams of Carbs.

444 Calories.

Deep Fried Eggs (1 Serving)

Ingredients:

2 Eggs

3 slices of Bacon

Directions:

1. Heat oil in your deep fryer to approximately 375 degrees.

2. Cook your bacon.

3. Crack eggs into your prep bowl.

4. Slip egg into the center of your fryer. Don't drop eggs in, try to slip the eggs in near the surface.

5. Using two different spatulas, corral your egg into a ball. This may take a little practice to get the hang of.

6. Fry for approximately 3-4 minutes or until bubbling stops.

7. Serve and Enjoy!

Nutritional Value:

27 grams of Protein.

24 grams of Fat.

1 gram of Carbs.

321 Calories.

Steak & Eggs (Serves 1)

Ingredients:

3 Eggs

1 tablespoon of Butter

4 ounces of Sirloin

1/4 of an Avocado

Pepper / Salt

Directions:

1. Melt butter in your pan. Fry the eggs until whites have been set and yolk is done to your desired preference. Season them with pepper and salt.

2. Cook sirloin in another pan until desired preference. Slice into small strips and season with pepper and salt.

3. Slice up avocado and add to your dish.

Nutritional Value:

44 grams of Protein.

26 grams of Fat.

3 grams of Carbs.

510 Calories.

Scotch Eggs (Serves 4)

Ingredients:

4 large Eggs

8 slices of Thick Cut Bacon

12 ounce package of Jimmy Dean's Pork Sausage

4 Toothpicks

Directions:

1. Hard boil your eggs.

2. Peel your eggs. Let them dry and cool off.

3. Split your sausage equally into four parts. Pat down each of these parts into a circle.

4. Place egg in each of these circles and wrap it with your sausage. Adjust your sausage so that your eggs are covered completely.

5. Refrigerate them for between approximately 30 to 60 minutes.

6. Form a cross out of two pieces of your bacon.

7. Place your wrapped egg in the center of the cross and fold your bacon over the egg. Use a toothpick to secure it together.

8. Repeat this process on all 4 eggs.

9. Cook eggs in a 450 degree convection oven for approximately 20 minutes. Regular ovens can work but it might need to be finished off using a broiler.

10. Eggs are done when your bacon is nice and crisp.

11. Serve and Enjoy!

<u>Nutritional Value - (Serving Size 1 Scotch Egg):</u>

25 grams of Protein.

33 grams of Fat.

2 grams of Carbs.

405 Calories.

One Skillet Eggs & Bacon

Ingredients:

4 large Eggs

8 slices of Bacon

1 tablespoon of Butter

1/2 cup of Chopped Cauliflower or Broccoli

1/2 cup of Finely Chopped Celery

1 Peeled Carrot

1/2 cup of Shredded Colby Jack Cheese

1/2 of a large Chopped White Onion.

Directions:

1. Slice your bacon across its grain into smaller strips.

2. Melt butter in a large sized skillet over medium heat.

3. Add your bacon and vegetables.

4. Stir often and saute your vegetables and bacon in the butter approximately 20 minutes. You want the bacon to start crisping on its edges and you want the vegetables to being caramelizing.

5. Spread your mixture over your skillet as evenly as possible and make four wells one in each quarter of the skillet.

6. Break an egg into each of the wells. Cook eggs until nearly done. Cook shorter if you like your yolks runny and longer if you like them harder.

7. When eggs are nearly done sprinkle cheese on top and let cook until cheese melts and eggs are done.

8. Serve and Enjoy!

Ricotta Scrambled Eggs (Serves 1)

Ingredients:

2 Eggs

150 grams of 2% Fat Ricotta Cheese

50 grams of Italian Dry Salami

1 teaspoon of Rosemary

1 tablespoon of Olive Oil

Pepper

Salt

Directions:

1. Chop your salami up into smaller cubes. Fry them together in a small pan using olive oil.

2. While frying, whisk your eggs, add pepper, rosemary, and salt.

3. Add your ricotta into egg mixture, mix well to break up any big lumps.

4. Add your eggs and ricotta mixture to the pan and cook for approximately 5 minutes until done.

5. Serve and Enjoy!

Nutritional Value:

28 grams of Protein.

45 grams of Fat.

5 grams of Carbs.

598 Calories.

Clouds of Eggs (Serves 4)

Ingredients:

4 large Eggs

2 slices of Bacon

2 tablespoons of Parmesan Cheese

Pepper

Salt

Onion Powder

Garlic Powder

Directions:

1. Split your egg yolks from your egg whites.

2. Cut up bacon and cook for some bacon bits.

3. Put your eggs in a bowl and then whip them till they are stiff.

4. Shred your Parmesan cheese into your egg whites and then add in bacon bits.

5. Split your egg white into four separate mounds on parchment paper or a silicon mat.

6. Bake your egg whites for 5 minutes at approximately 350 degrees until they are set. 7. Put egg yolk into each of your mounds.

8. Bake your egg whites until brown.

9. Serve and Enjoy!

Nutritional Value - (Serving Size 1 Egg):

6 grams of Protein.

7 grams of Fat.

1 gram of Carbs.

98 Calories.

Low-Carb Sausage & Egg Muffin (Serves 1)

Ingredients:

Muffin

1 Egg

1 tablespoon Almond Milk

1 tablespoon Coconut Flour

1/2 tablespoon Olive Oil

1/2 teaspoon Baking Powder

1 pinch of Salt

Filling

1 Egg

1 slice of Cheese

1 Sausage Link

1/4 teaspoon of Thyme

1/4 teaspoon of Salt

1/4 teaspoon of Sage

1/8 teaspoon of Black Pepper

Directions:

1. Preheat oven to 400 degrees.

2. To make low carb muffin, crack your egg into your mixing bowl and add each of the muffin ingredients.

3. Mix well. Get rid of clumps and pour your batter into a ramekin. Bake approximately 15 minutes.

4. Crack egg into your ramekin, give egg a good stir and season with both salt and pepper. Bake approximately 10 minutes.

5. Cut open a pork sausage link and discard its casing. You can also use an actual breakfast sausage.

6. Add seasonings to your sausage meat and mix using your hands. Shape them into a patty and then cook using a hot pan for 4 to 5 minutes on both sides.

7. Once finished, take out of the oven and cut your muffins into some thin halves. Toast them until they are browned.

8. Put together your sandwich and add your slice of cheese.

Nutritional Value:

29 grams of Protein.

37 grams of Fat.

3 grams of Carbs.

460 Calories.

Cali Chicken Omelet (Serves 1)

Ingredients:

2 slices of Bacon (Chopped and Cooked)

2 Eggs

1 ounce of Deli Cut Chicken

1/4 of an Avocado

1 tablespoon of Mayo

1 Campari Tomato

1 teaspoon of Mustard

Directions:

1. Crack your eggs and beat them in a small bowl. Add to hot pan. Pull sides of eggs towards the center to cook your omelet faster. Season them with pepper and salt.

2. Once eggs are half cooked (approximately 5 minutes), add your bacon, chicken, tomato, and sliced avocado. Also, add in your mayo and mustard.

3. Fold your omelet over onto itself. Cover using a lid. Cook until finished (approximately 5 minutes).

4. Serve and Enjoy!

Nutritional Value:

25 grams of Protein.

32 grams of Fat.

4 grams of net Carbs.

415 Calories.

Breakfast Lettuce Taco (Serves 2)

Ingredients:

4 large Eggs

2 Romaine Lettuce Leafs

2 tablespoons of Heavy Cream

6 slices of Bacon

2 slices of Cheddar Cheese

2 tablespoons of Shredded Cheddar

Pepper

Salt

Onion Powder

Directions:

1. Cook your bacon to desired preference.

2. Whisk your eggs, cream, and add seasonings.

3. Scramble the eggs and mix in the cheese at the end.

4. Combine your eggs, cheese, bacon, and lettuce.

5. Serve and Enjoy!

Nutritional Value - (Serving Size 1 Taco):

29 grams of Protein.

40 grams of Fat.

3 grams of Carbs.

499 Calories.

Pesto & Feta Omelet (Serves 1)

Ingredients:

3 Eggs

1 tablespoon of Butter

1 tablespoon of Heavy Cream

1 ounce of Feta Cheese

1 tablespoon of Pesto

Pepper

Salt

Directions:

1. Melt tablespoon of your butter in the pan and let it heat up.

2. Beat eggs in bowl with a tablespoon of heavy cream.

3. Pour eggs into a hot pan and cook until nearly done.

4. Sprinkle feta cheese on half of omelet. Spread a tablespoon of pesto on the same half.

5. Fold omelet over onto itself. Cook for approximately 4 to 5 minutes so that feta cheese all melts and your eggs cook properly.

6. Garnish with more feta cheese on top.

7. Serve and Enjoy!

Nutritional Value:

30 grams of Protein.

46 gram of Fat.

2.5 grams of Carbs.

570 Calories.

Breakfast Keto Pizza (Serves 2)

Ingredients:

4 Eggs

2 ounces of Cheddar Cheese

4 slices of Bacon

10 slices of Pepperoni

Pepper

Salt

Garlic Powder

Onion Powder

Directions:

1. Cook your bacon and reserve your bacon grease in the skillet.

2. Let your pan cool a bit.

3. Crack eggs into your pan and put them all close together.

4. Apply your seasoning.

5. Cook at 450 degrees in your oven for approximately 6 minutes.

6. Add toppings and cheddar.

7. Cook for 4 more minutes.

8. Put the bacon on top.

9. Serve and Enjoy!

Nutritional Value - (Serving Size 1/2 of Pizza):

22 grams of Protein.

24 grams of Fat.

1 gram of Carbs.

307 Calories.

Spicy Shrimp Omelet (Serves 2)

Ingredients:

6 Eggs

10 large Shrimp

1 handful of Spinach

4 Grape Tomatoes

1/4 of an Onion

1 teaspoon of Cayenne

1 tablespoon of Sriracha Salt

1 Sprig of Parsley

Directions:

1. Chop your onion and slice your grape tomatoes lengthwise in half.

2. Fire pan to medium heat. Add your onions and salt. Add the grape tomatoes cut side down so they can roast a little bit.

3. When your onions get translucent add in spinach and let it shrink and wilt enough for some of your shrimp to fit in.

4. Throw the shrimp in.

5. Crack each egg leaving room for all of them. Take your spoon and jiggle around the whites so they grab everything that is underneath them.

6. Place a lid on your pan. Let omelet cook for approximately 6 to 8 minutes. Watch your eggs, once thin film of white has covered the yolks they're ready. If eggs are still runny let them cook a bit longer.

7. Once omelet is done, run your knife across each of the yolks and let them ooze out onto your whole omelet. Garnish with your parsley.

8. Serve and Enjoy!

Nutritional Value:

36 grams of Protein.

17 grams of Fat.

4 grams of Carbs.

329 Calories.

Cast Iron Skillet Frittata (Serves 8)

Ingredients:

12 Eggs

1 small Pepper

1 small Onion

8 slices of Bacon

12 ounces of Cheddar Cheese

1 head of Cauliflower

542 grams of Brussels Sprouts

6 ounces of Heavy Cream

1/2 teaspoon of Onion Powder

1/2 teaspoon of Garlic Powder

1/2 teaspoon of Pepper

1/2 teaspoon of Salt

Directions:

1. Cook bacon until it's crisp. Keep your bacon grease in your skillet.

2. Thinly slice your pepper and onion.

3. Shred your cauliflower and Brussels sprouts.

4. Cook vegetables in your skillet.

5. While veggies are cooking, prepare your egg mixture with eggs, cream, and spices. Whisk them to combine.

6. When vegetables are finished. Should be translucent and cooked. Crumble and add in your cheese and bacon.

7. Mix well together and add in your eggs. Mix again.

8. Cook 2 to 3 minutes on stove top.

9. Transfer over to skillet and cook in your oven for 25 minutes at 450 degrees.

10. Take out of oven and slice.

11. Serve and Enjoy!

Nutritional Value - (Serving Size 1/8 of Frittata):

29 grams of Protein.

35 grams of Fat.

18 grams of Carbs.

491 Calories.

Cajun Hash (Serves 2)

Ingredients:

2 tablespoons of Ghee or Olive Oil

1/2 of an Onion

1 Egg

2 tablespoons of Minced Garlic

1 pound bag of Frozen Cauliflower (chopped into even sized small chunks)

1 teaspoon of Cajun Seasoning

1/2 of a Green Pepper (chopped into 1/4 inch slices)

8 ounces of Shaved Red Pastrami (chopped into 1-inch slices)

Directions:

1. In your ghee or olive oil, saute chopped onions approximately 5 minutes on medium heat.

2. After 5 minutes, saute garlic for approximately 2 minutes.

3. Squeeze out any excess water from chopped cauliflower. Add it to your saute and cook for 5 to 10 minutes. It will be done once it's crispy and brown.

4. Add your Cajun seasoning and mix in.

5. Add your green peppers and chopped pastrami.

6. Toss and cook till it's hot all around. Should take approximately 5 minutes.

7. Add to a bowl.

8. Fry an egg sunny side up, add to the top of your hash, then dash with Cajun seasoning.

9. Serve and Enjoy!

Bacon Hash (Serves 2)

Ingredients:

4 Eggs

6 slices of Bacon

Jalapeno Slices

1 small Onion

1 small Pepper

Directions:

1. Slice your onion and pepper into a thin strip.

2. Dice your jalapeno slices up as small as you can.

3. Fry all the vegetables in your cast iron pan.

4. Remove when the vegetables are browning and translucent.

5. Chop your bacon using a food processor until it's broken in chunks. Don't overdo it. You don't want it to be a paste.

6. Mix everything together.

7. Cook your hash until bacon is about to crisp.

8. Fry an egg.

9. Arrange it on your plate and top it with your fried egg.

10. Serve and Enjoy!

Nutritional Value - (Serving Size 2 Eggs):

23 grams of Protein.

24 grams of Fat.

11 grams of Carbs.

366 Calories.

Fried Crusty Cheddar (Serves 1)

Ingredients:

1 Egg

2 slices of Cheddar Cheese

1 teaspoon of Ground Flaxseed

1 teaspoon of Almond Flour

1 teaspoon of Hemp Nuts

1 tablespoon of Olive Oil

Pepper

Salt

Directions:

1. Heat olive oil in your frying pan over medium heat.

2. Whisk your egg with pepper and salt.

3. Mix your flaxseed with hemp nuts and almond flour.

4. Coat your cheddar slices with your egg mixture and then with your dry mixture.

5. Fry them for approximately 3 minutes on both sides.

6. Serve and Enjoy!

Nutritional Value:

35 grams of Protein.

48 grams of Fat.

5 grams of Carbs.

588 Calories.

Onion & Cheese Quiche - (Makes 2 Quiches or 12 Servings)

Ingredients:

12 large Organic Eggs

5 to 6 cups of Shredded Colby Jack Cheese or Muenster Cheese

1 White Onion - large and finely chopped

2 tablespoons of Butter

2 cups of Heavy Cream

2 teaspoons of Dried Thyme

1 teaspoon of Salt

1 teaspoon of Ground Black Pepper

Directions:

1. Prepare your oven to 350 degrees.

2. In a large skillet add your butter and melt over a medium-low heat.

3. Add your vegetables and saute until your onions are soft and translucent.

4. Remove them from the heat and allow to cool.

5. Butter two of your deep pie pans or 10-inch quiche pans. Put in 2 cups of your shredded cheese to cover the bottom of each of your buttered pans.

6. Add 1/2 of your cooled vegetable mixture to each one of the pans. Make sure they are evenly layered over the cheese.

7. Crack all of your eggs and pour them into your large mixing bowl.

8. Add your spices and cream together. Whisk till frothy and well mixed.

9. Pour 1/2 of your mixture over each pan and use a fork to evenly distribute the cheese and veggies into your egg and cream mix.

10. Slide pans into your oven. Leave about an inch between the pans. Continue to bake for 20 to 25 minutes. Should be slightly golden colored in the middle and puffy looking. Test by sticking a knife in the center. If it comes out clean it means they are finished.

11. Remove from oven and cut each of your quiches into 6 servings of equal size.

12. You can either serve immediately or cool in the fridge. Will stay good for about a week refrigerated and about two weeks when in the freezer.

13. Serve and Enjoy!

Nutritional Value: (Serving Size is 1/6 of a quiche.)

16 grams of Protein.

33 grams of Fat.

4 grams of Carbs.

382 Calories.

Chicken Fajita Quiche (16 Slices)

Ingredients:

24 large Egg Whites

1 package of McCormick Gluten-Free Taco Seasoning Mix

2 medium Bell Peppers (steamed & diced)

12 ounces of Grilled Chicken Breast (diced)

Directions:

1. Preheat oven to 300 degrees. Lightly coat two 9-inch round baking pans using a nonstick cooking spray.

2. In a large bowl, whisk egg whites together with taco seasoning mix. Stir in your chicken and bell peppers. Equally divide mixture between two baking pans.

3. Bake for around 25 to 30 minutes. You don't want the center to move when it's shaken slightly.

4. Let cool in your pan for 10 minutes before slicing each of the quiches into 8 pieces each.

5. Serve and Enjoy!

Nutritional Value - (Serving Size 2 Slices):

20.5 grams of Protein.

2.3 grams of Fat.

6 grams of Carbs.

128 Calories.

Ricotta Cheese w/ Vanilla (Serves 1)

Ingredients:

200 grams of 2% Fat Ricotta Cheese

1 sachet of Vanilla Flavoring

1 tablespoon of Creme Fraiche

Directions:

1. Mix your ricotta with your creme fraiche and vanilla flavoring.

2. Serve and Enjoy!

Nutritional Value:

8 grams of Protein.

18 grams of Fat.

3 grams of Carbs.

290 Calories.

Breakfast Chorizo Casserole (Serves 10)

Ingredients:

12 Eggs

1 small Onion

1 small Pepper

16 ounces of Ground Chorizo

366 grams of Spinach

12 tablespoons of Heavy Cream

1 teaspoon of Garlic Powder

1 teaspoon of Salt

1 teaspoon of Pepper

1 teaspoon of Onion Powder

9 ounces of Cherry Tomatoes

8 ounces of Cheddar

Directions:

1. Cook your spinach in the microwave.

2. Chop or grind up your chorizo and then cook in your skillet until it is browned.

3. Place finished chorizo in a big bowl.

4. Thinly slice pepper and onion. Cook them in the same skillet. Place in a large bowl when finished.

5. Add finished spinach to the bowl.

6. Whisk together your eggs, spices, and heavy cream.

7. Add your cheese to your bowl and then combine. Add egg mixture.

8. Transfer to your greased casserole dish.

9. Add cherry tomatoes.

10. Cook for 50 minutes at approximately 350 degrees.

11. Remove from oven.

12. Serve and Enjoy!

Nutritional Value: - (Serving Size 1/10 of Casserole)

24 grams of Protein.

28 grams of Fat.

7 grams of Carbs.

362 Calories.

Two Cheese Muffins (Makes 15 Muffins)

Ingredients:

2 Eggs

2 cups of Almond Flour

1/4 teaspoon of Salt

1/2 teaspoon of Baking Soda

1/2 teaspoon of Dried Thyme

1 cup of Sour Cream

1 cup of Shredded Cheddar

1/2 cup of Shredded Muenster

1/8 cup of Melted Butter

Directions:

1. Preheat your oven to 400 degrees. Place your cupcake papers in each muffin hole on a normal size 12 count muffin pan.

2. Whisk your dry ingredients and almond flour together.

3. In a different bowl, lightly beat your eggs and mix in the butter and sour cream.

4. Add your liquid mixture to almond flour mix. If batter seems a little too thick add a tablespoon of heavy cream or water.

5. Add your cheese and stir in until it is distributed evenly.

6. Spoon your mixture into the muffin cups. Each should be filled 3/4 of the way.

7. Bake for approximately 5 minutes at 400 degrees.

8. Turn down your oven temperature to 350 degrees and bake it for another 20 minutes or until it is golden.

9. Take out and let it cool down.

10. Serve and Enjoy!

Nutritional Value - (1 Muffin)

6 grams of Protein.

15 grams of Fat.

5 grams of Carbs.

166 Calories.

Sour Cream Blueberry Muffins (Makes 15 Muffins)

Ingredients:

2 Eggs

2 cups of Almond Flour

1 cup of Sour Cream

1/4 cup of Erythritol

1/2 teaspoon of Salt

1/2 teaspoon of Baking Soda

1/8 cup of Melted Butter

4 ounces of Fresh Blueberries

Directions

1. Preheat your oven to 350 degrees. Put cupcake papers in each muffin hole of your 12 count muffin pan. You'll want to use two of these pans as the recipe will produce 15 muffins.

2. Whisk you dry ingredients and almond flour together.

3. In a different bowl, lightly beat eggs and then mix in your butter and sour cream till smooth.

4. Add the almond flour mix and sour cream mix together and stir well.

5. Add in your blueberries and stir until they are distributed evenly.

6. Spoon your mixture in each of the muffin cups. Fill them 1/2 full.

7. Bake for approximately 20 minutes. Are done when golden.

8. Let cool off.

9. Serve and Enjoy!

Nutritional Value - (1 Muffin)

5 grams of Protein.

13 grams of Fat.

5 grams of Carbs.

147 Calories.

Raspberry Protein Pancakes

Ingredients:

1/4 cup of Egg Whites

1/2 of a Banana

1 scoop of Whey Protein Powder

2 tablespoons of Almond Milk

1 tablespoon of Cinnamon

2 tablespoons of Greek Yogurt

1 tablespoon of Chia Seeds

3/4 cup of Raspberries

Directions :

1. Mash up banana.

2. Grind up chia seeds.

3. Add all your ingredients except the raspberries to your bowl and stir together well.

4. Add your raspberries and stir.

5. Spray your small pan with some olive oil spray and then pour in your mix.

6. Cook pancakes on medium heat until your edges are brown. Once this occurs flip your pancakes.

7. Continue cooking until the middle has been well cooked. Check with a fork.

8. Add to a plate along with your Greek yogurt.

9. Serve and Enjoy!

Nutritional Value

36 grams of Protein.

1 gram of Fat.

29 grams of Carbs.

275 Calories.

Keto Bacon Pancakes (Makes 8 Pancakes)

Ingredients:

1 Egg

8 slices of Bacon

1 cup of Carbquik

1/4 cup of Water

1/2 cup of Heavy Cream

1/2 cup of Melted Unsalted Butter

1 tablespoon of Sugar-Free Vanilla Syrup

1/2 teaspoon of Baking Soda

Directions:

1. Cook your bacon.

2. Melt your butter in a microwave.

3. Mix together baking soda and Carbquik.

4. Add your liquid ingredients and mix it all together.

5. Heat your pan over a medium-high heat. Spray it with Pam.

6. Spoon some batter onto pan. Don't make the pancake so large you can't flip it. Add your bacon.

7. When edges brown or bubbles form in center flip your pancake.

8. Continue to cook for another minute until center is cooked. Check with a fork.

9. Remove pancakes and make next one.

10. Repeat process until all your pancakes are finished.

10. Serve and Enjoy!

Nutritional Value: - (Serving Size 2 Pancakes)

12 grams of Protein.

46 grams of Fat.

5 grams of Carbs.

443 Calories.

Pumpkin Cream Cheese Pancakes (1 Serving - Makes 2 Pancakes)

Ingredients:

Pancake List:

2 Eggs

2 ounces of Cream Cheese

2 tablespoons of Coconut Flour

1/4 tablespoon of Pumpkin Pie Spice

Pumpkin Butter List:

3 tablespoons of Unsalted Butter

1/2 tablespoon of 100% Pumpkin

1/16 teaspoon of Raw Stevia

Directions:

1. Start with pumpkin butter. Mix together pumpkin and butter. Microwave for intervals of 10 seconds until it is smooth. Once it's smooth, add in your Stevia for taste.

2. Next work on pancakes. Mix your eggs, cream cheese, pumpkin pie spice, and coconut flour until blended together.

3. Heat a non-stick pan over medium heat. Add a tablespoon of butter.

4. When butter begins to brown add in half of your pancake mix.

5. Once edges brown or the center bubbles, flip your pancake.

6. Cook for around another minute until center is cooked. Check with your fork.

7. Remove from pan and add to your plate.

8. Repeat process with next pancake.

9. Once pancakes are all done add your pumpkin butter.

10. Serve and Enjoy!

Squash Spaghetti Pancakes (Serves 2)

Ingredients:

2 Eggs

4 slices of Thick Cut Bacon

10 ounces of Cooked Spaghetti Squash

1 ounce of Parmesan Cheese

1 teaspoon of Garlic Powder

1 teaspoon of Pepper

1 teaspoon of Salt

1 teaspoon of Onion Powder

Directions:

1. Cook your spaghetti squash.

2. Cook bacon until it's crispy.

3. Add your eggs, spices, cheese, and spaghetti squash to bowl and mix.

4. Crumble your bacon and add it to your mixture.

5. Heat your bacon grease in the skillet until they are shimmering.

6. Scoop your mixture into bacon grease. Make four piles and then use a spatula to compress your piles flat.

7. After bottom begins to brown flip it.

8. You can add a dollop of sour cream or some chives if you want.

9. Serve and Enjoy!

Nutritional Value - (Serving Size 2 Pancakes):

19 grams of Protein.

18 grams of Fat.

10 grams of Carbs.

287 Calories.

Crunchy Keto Cereal w/ Strawberries

Ingredients:

1 package of Bob's Red Mill Flaked Coconut

Unsweetened Almond Milk

Ground Cinnamon

2 medium sized Strawberries

Stevia

Parchment Paper or Coconut Oil

Directions:

1. Preheat oven to 350 degrees.

2. Line your cookie sheet with parchment paper. If no parchment paper grease your cook sheet using coconut oil.

3. Pour coconut flakes on cookie sheet.

4. Cook in your oven for 5 minutes.

5. Shuffle flakes around and continue cooking till they are a lightly toasted and lightly tan.

6. Take flakes out of your oven.

7. Sprinkle them lightly with cinnamon. Can also sprinkle lightly with Stevia.

8. Throw your toasted chips in a bowl and pour your almond milk over them.

9. Slice up two strawberries as the garnish on top.

10. Serve and Enjoy!

Keto French Toast (Serves 4)

Ingredients:

8 large Eggs

2 teaspoon of Baking Powder

1 tablespoon of Swerve or Sugar Equivalent

1/4 cup of Coconut Flour

2 grams of Salt

3/4 cup of Unsweetened Almond Milk

1 teaspoon of Vanilla Extract

1/4 cup of Melted Butter

1/2 cup of Heavy Whipping Cream

1/4 cup of Fresh Whole Butter

Directions:

1. Mix your coconut flour, baking powder, salt, and sugar.

2. In a different bowl, whisk together 4 of your 8 eggs. Add 1/4 cup of your almond milk and vanilla. Whisk together.

3. Add your dry and wet ingredients together and whisk. Continue to do so while pouring in melted butter.

4. Grease your 12 microwave safe containers. Use wide containers.

5. Microwave muffins. For each additional muffin add a minute to microwave time. I made 2 batches of 6 muffins with 6 minutes for each batch.

6. While muffins are cooking, in a large mixing bowl, whisk together your other 4 eggs, 1/2 cup of heavy cream, and 1/2 cup of almond milk.

7. As muffins come out of your microwave, pop them out of containers and allow them to cool for a minute. When they are cool enough, add to your egg mixture and let them sit for a couple minutes. Flip them occasionally while letting them sit.

8. Once they've absorbed some of the mixture, heat up a large skillet over medium-low heat. Add some fresh butter and melt it.

9. Fry your muffins like you would French toast.

10. Serve and Enjoy!

Nutritional Value - (Serving Size 1 Piece of French Toast):

16 grams of Protein.

44 grams of Fat.

8 grams of Carbs.

491 Calories.

Breakfast Peanut Butter Bars (Serves 12)

Ingredients:

2 Egg Whites

1 cup of Chunky Peanut Butter

1/2 cup of Flaxseed Meal

1/2 cup of Sweetener

1/2 cup of Almond Meal

1/2 cup of Sugar-Free Chocolate Chips

1/2 cup of Almonds

1/2 cup of Cashews

1/2 teaspoon of Chia Seeds

Directions:

1. Preheat your oven to 350 degrees. Line your 8 x 8 pan or dish with parchment paper.

2. In a big bowl mix together all your ingredients until they are well combined.

3. Pour your mixture into pan and press mixture into the pan so that it's flat.

4. Bake for approximately 10 to 15 minutes.

5. Let cool down and refrigerate for approximately 30 minutes.

6. Cut into 12 equal size bars.

7. Keep bars refrigerated they are being served.

8. Serve and Enjoy!

Nutritional Value - (Serving Size 1 Bar):

11 grams of Protein.

23 grams of Fat.

15 grams of Carbs.

305 Calories.

Snickerdoodle Crepes (Serves 8)

Ingredients:

Crepes

6 Eggs

5 ounces of Softened Cream Cheese

1 teaspoon of Cinnamon

1 tablespoon of Sugar Substitute.

Butter

Filling

8 tablespoons of Softened Butter

1 tablespoon of Cinnamon

1/3 cup of Granulated Sugar Substitute

Directions:

1. Blend all your crepe ingredients together except for the butter. Place them in a blender or your magic bullet until they are smooth. Let batter rest for approximately 5 minutes.

2. Heat your butter in a non-stick pan over medium heat until it is sizzling. Pour in enough batter to form a 6-inch crepe. Proceed to cook for approximately 2 minutes before flipping and cooking the other side for an additional minute. Remove crepe and place on a warm plate. This should make about 8 crepes.

3. In a small bowl, mix together cinnamon and sweetener until they are combined. Stir half of this mixture into the softened butter until it is smooth.

4. Spread a tablespoon of butter mixture in the middle of the crepe. Roll it up and sprinkle and additional teaspoon of mixture onto it.

5. Serve and Enjoy!

Nutritional Value - (Serving Size 1 Crepe):

12 grams of Protein.

42 grams of Fat.

2 grams of Carbs.

434 Calories.

Breakfast Chia Bowl (Serves 2)

Ingredients:

2 cups of Unsweetened NonDairy Milk

1/4 cup of Whole Chia Seeds

2 tablespoons of Pure Maple Syrup

1 teaspoon of Vanilla Extract

Toppings

Fresh Fruit

Nuts (optional)

Cinnamon (optional)

Directions:

1. Combine your milk, seeds, vanilla, and syrup in the bowl and stir it all together.

2. Let stand for 30 minutes. Whisk together to keep seeds from getting clumped together. Move to air tight container. Cover and refrigerate overnight.

3. Divide between 2 different bowls and serve with your choice of toppings.

Nutritional Value - (Without Any Toppings):

14 grams of Protein.

15 grams of Fat.

35 grams of Carbs.

298 Calories.

Almond Bacon Waffles (Serves 2)

Ingredients:

2 Eggs

4 slices of Bacon

3/4 cup of Almond Flour

5 tablespoons of Melted Unsalted Butter

1 1/2 teaspoons of Baking Soda

1 1/2 teaspoons of Splenda

Directions:

1. Cook you bacon until it's crisp.

2. Place eggs in warm water to get them heated up.

3. Mix dry ingredients. This includes Splenda, baking powder, and almond flour.

4. Add 2 eggs and mix well.

5. Microwave your butter and add it to the mix.

6. Preheat your waffle maker.

7. Once heated spray with Pam and fill with batter. Add in your bacon.

8. Cook waffle. Follow your waffle maker's instructions. Many will vary on time and temperature.

9. Remove waffle and add any desired toppings.

10. Serve and Enjoy!

Nutritional Value - (Serving Size 1 Waffle):

21 grams of Protein.

61 grams of Fat.

10 grams of Carbs.

648 Calories.

Keto Pumpkin Bread Loaf (10 Slices)

Ingredients:

3 large Egg Whites

1 1/2 cup of Almond Flour

1/2 cup of Pumpkin Puree

1/4 cup of Swerve Sweetener

1/2 cup of Coconut Milk

1/4 cup of Psyllium Husk Powder

2 teaspoons of Baking Powder

1/2 teaspoon of Kosher Salt

1 1/2 teaspoons of Pumpkin Pie Spice

Directions:

1. Measure dry ingredients into your sifter.

2. Sift ingredients into a big bowl.

3. Preheat over to 350 degrees. Fill a 9 x 9 baking dish with a cup of water and put on bottom rack of your oven.

4. Add coconut milk to your bowl and mix together.

5. Whip your egg whites in a different bowl.

6. Fold in 1/3 of eggs whites to your dough mixture so moisture gets absorbed. Add rest of your egg whites and fold them gently into dough.

7. Grease a bread loaf pan with coconut oil or butter. Spread out your dough into bread pan.

8. Bake for approximately 75 minutes.

9. Remove from oven and allow to cool.

10. Slice into 10 equal pieces.

11. Serve and Enjoy!

Nutritional Value - (Serving Size 1 Slice):

4.5 grams of Protein.

8.7 grams of Fats.

3.1 grams of Carbs.

120 Calories.

Coconut Blueberry Porridge (2 Servings)

Ingredients:

Porridge

1/4 cup of Ground Flaxseed

1 cup of Almond Milk

1/4 cup of Coconut Flour

1 teaspoon of Cinnamon

10 drops of Liquid Stevia

1 teaspoon of Vanilla Extract

Pinch of Salt

Toppings

2 tablespoons of Butter

60 grams of Blueberries

2 tablespoons of Pumpkin Seeds

1 ounce of Shaved Coconut

Directions:

1. Place a cup of almond milk over a low heat.

2. Add in your flaxseed, salt, cinnamon, and coconut flour. Whisk to break any clumps.

3. Heat until bubbling slightly. Add your vanilla extract and liquid Stevia.

4. When the mixture is thick turn off your flame and add in toppings.

5. Serve and Enjoy!

Nutritional Value:

10 grams of Protein.

34 grams of Fat.

8 grams of Carbs.

405 Calories.

Cream, Flaxseed, & Goji Cup (Serves 1)

Ingredients:

30 grams of Ground Flaxseed

100 milliliters of 35% Fat Cooking Cream

1 teaspoon of Dark Unsweetened Cocoa Powder

1 tablespoon of Goji Berries

Freshly Brewed Coffee

Liquid Sweetener

Directions:

1. Mix your ground flaxseed, cream, and cocoa until flaxseed is covered. Add liquid sweetener for more sweetness.

2. Add coffee. If you don't like coffee add a couple spoons worth of water.

3. Add Goji berries.

4. Serve and Enjoy!

Nutritional Value:

7 grams of Protein.

42 grams of Fat.

10 grams of Carbs.

441 Calories.

Lemon Blueberry Muffins (Makes 15 Muffins)

Ingredients:

2 Eggs

1 cup of Heavy Cream

2 cups of Almond Flour

1/8 cup of Melted Butter

4 oz of Fresh Blueberries

1/2 teaspoon of Baking Soda

5 packets of Stevia or Splenda

1/2 teaspoon of Lemon Flavoring or Extract

1/4 teaspoon of Salt

1/2 teaspoon of Dried Lemon Zest

Directions:

1. Preheat your oven 350 degrees. Place some cupcake paper in each muffin hole of a normal sized 12 serving muffin pan. This recipe will make 15 muffins so you'll need two pans.

2. Mix cream and almond flour.

3. Add in your eggs one by one. Stir until they are all mixed.

4. Add sweetener, butter, spices, flavoring, and baking soda. Mix together.

5. Add your blueberries. Stir till they are all distributed evenly.

6. Spoon your mixture into the pans. Fill each spot until it is 1/2 full.

7. Bake around 20 minutes. Should be golden colored when finished.

8. Take out of your oven and let cool off.

9. Serve and Enjoy!

Nutritional Value - (1 muffin)

5 grams of Protein.

17 grams of Fat.

6 grams of Carbs.

184 Calories.

Low-Carb Blueberry Muffins (Serves 6)

Ingredients:

3 large Organic Eggs

1/4 cup of Heavy Cream

5 tablespoons of Organic Coconut Flour

1/3 cup of Erythritol Crystals

1/2 cup of Frozen Organic Blueberries

Directions:

1. Preheat oven to 350 degrees.

2. Line your muffin pan with some paper liners.

3. In a big bowl, add eggs, erythritol, and cream. Whisk together until it is mixed well.

4. Add coconut flour to your egg mix and whisk until it is smooth.

5. Let rest for 5 minutes until your batter thickens. Add your frozen blueberries and mix in well.

6. Scoop batter into your muffin cups.

7. Bake for approximately 25 to 30 minutes.

8. Allow to cool.

9. Serve and Enjoy!

Nutritional Value - (Serving Size 1 Muffin):

5.6 grams of Protein.

7.9 grams of Fat.

2.6 grams of Carbs.

105 Calories.

Cinnamon Instant Oatmeal

Ingredients:

2/3 cup of Chia Seeds

2/3 cup of Unsweetened Coconut

2/3 cup of Golden Flax Meal

2 tablespoons of Ground Cinnamon

1/2 cup of Hot Water

2 tablespoons of Unsweetened Coconut Milk

Sweetener

Directions:

1. Combine your golden flax meal, chia seed, cinnamon, and unsweetened coconut in an airtight container.

2. Scoop out 1/2 cup of this mixture and keep rest stored in a container.

3. Pour 1/2 cup of water on your mixture and allow to sit between 3 and 5 minutes.

4. Add sweetener and coconut milk into your bowl. Stir to combine.

5. Serve and Enjoy!

Gluten Free Banana Bread (Serves 8)

Ingredients:

Wet Ingredients

3 Ripe Bananas

1/4 cup of Honey

1 Juiced Orange

Pinch of Orange Zest

1/4 teaspoon of Vanilla Extract

2 tablespoons of Coconut Oil

Dry Ingredients

1/2 teaspoon of Salt

1 1/3 cup of Almond Flour

3/4 teaspoon of Cinnamon

1/8 teaspoon of Cayenne

1/2 teaspoon of Baking Soda

1 teaspoon of Xanthan Gum

1 teaspoon of Baking Powder

Fold-Ins

2 Grated Carrots

3/4 cup of Chopped Walnuts

3/ cup of Flaxseeds

1/4 teaspoon of Grated Fresh Ginger

Topping

Coconut Butter

Honey

Directions:

1. Preheat your oven to 410 degrees.

2. Mash bananas until they are in a thick wet mush.

3. Take zest from the peel of your orange. Cut in half and juice the whole thing into your bananas.

4. Add vanilla extract, honey, and coconut oil.

5. Add in all your dry ingredients.

6. Shred ginger carrots to fold in. Chop walnuts and throw them into your mixture.

7. Fold in rest of your ingredients.

8. Grease medium 8 x 4 bread pan with butter or coconut oil. Pour in your batter.

9. Bake for approximately 25 minutes at 410 degrees. Lower to 350 degrees and bake for another 30 minutes.

10. Let bread cool. Drizzle honey on top. Slice into 8 pieces.

11. Serve and Enjoy!

Nutritional Value - (Serving Size 1 Slice of Bread)

8 grams of Protein.

24 grams of Fat.

23 grams of Carbs.

357 Calories.

Morning Detox Tea (Serves 1)

Ingredients:

1 cup of Warm Water

2 tablespoons of Apple Cider Vinegar

1 tablespoon of Honey

2 tablespoons of Lemon Juice

1 dash of Cayenne

1 teaspoon of Cinnamon

Directions:

1. Combine all your ingredients and stir well.

2. Serve and Enjoy!

Nutritional Value:

0 grams of Protein.

0 grams of Fat.

20 grams of Carbs.

84 Calories.

High Fiber Coffee & Coconut Cup (1 Serving)

Ingredients:

30 grams of Ground Flaxseed

30 grams of Unsweetened Ground Flaxseed

1 tablespoon of Coconut Oil

1/2 cup of Unsweetened Black Coffee

Liquid Sweetener

Directions:

1. Mix flaxseed and coconut flakes together well.

2. Add coconut oil. Pour hot coffee on it and mix. Adjust level of thickness by adding more still water or coffee.

3. Add 3 to 4 drops of liquid sweetener.

4. Serve and Enjoy!

Nutritional Value:

4 grams of Protein.

27 grams of Fat.

7 grams of Carbs.

277 Calories.

Heavenly Chocolate Milk - (Makes 2 Servings)

Ingredients:

16 oz of Unsweetened Almond Milk

4 oz of Heavy Cream

Stevia or Low-Carb Sweetener

1 scoop of Whey Chocolate Isolate Powder.

* 1/2 cup of Crushed Ice. Optional if you want your drink to be thicker. Will also have a less intense flavor.

Directions:

1. Put each of your ingredients in a blender.

2. Blend until it is smooth.

3. Serve and Enjoy!

Nutritional Value:

15 grams of Protein.

25 grams of Fat.

4 grams of Carbs.

292 Calories.

Iced Matcha Latte (Serves 1)

Ingredients:

1 tablespoon of Coconut Oil

1 cup of Unsweetened Cashew Milk

1 teaspoon of Matcha Powder

1/8 teaspoon of Vanilla Bean

2 Ice Cubes

Directions:

1. Combine all your ingredients in your blender and continue to blend until your ice cubes are broken up.

2. Sprinkle some extra matcha on top as the garnish.

3. Serve and Enjoy!

Nutritional Value:

1 gram of Protein.

15 grams of Fat.

0.5 grams of Carbs.

148 Calories.

Strawberry Almond Milk - (Makes 2 Servings)

Ingredients:

16 oz of Unsweetened Almond Milk

4 oz of Heavy Cream

1/4 cup of Unsweetened Frozen Strawberries

Stevia or Low-Carb Sweetener

1 scoop of Whey Vanilla Isolate Powder

Directions:

1. Put each of your ingredients in a blender.

2. Blend until it is smooth.

3. Serve and Enjoy!

Nutritional Value:

15 grams of Protein.

25 grams of Fat.

7 grams of Carbs.

304 Calories.

Blueberry Almond Milk - (Makes 2 Servings)

Ingredients:

16 oz of Unsweetened Almond Milk

4 oz of Heavy Cream

1/4 cup of Unsweetened Frozen Blueberries

Stevia or Low-Carb Sweetener

1 scoop of Whey Vanilla Isolate Powder.

Directions:

1. Put each of your ingredients in a blender.

2. Blend until it is smooth.

3. Serve and Enjoy!

Nutritional Value:

15 grams of Protein.

25 grams of Fat.

6 grams of Carbs.

302 Calories.

Orange Cooler Creamsicle - (Makes 2 Servings)

Ingredients:

16 ounces of Unsweetened Almond Milk

4 ounces of Heavy Cream

1/4 cup of Unsweetened Frozen Blueberries

Stevia or Low-Carb Sweetener

1 scoop of Whey Dreamsicle Powder

* 1/2 cup of Crushed Ice. Optional if you want your drink to be thicker. Will also have a less intense flavor

Directions:

1. Put each of your ingredients in a blender.

2. Blend until it is smooth.

3. Serve and Enjoy!

Nutritional Value:

15 grams of Protein.

25 grams of Fat.

4 grams of Carbs.

290 Calories.

Chapter Seven: Ketogenic Diet Lunch Recipes

In this section, I will give you 50 ketogenic lunch recipes you can make yourself. I'll include both basic recipes and a few more advanced recipes. That way no matter what your level in the kitchen you'll be able to prepare healthy low carb keto meals to keep you on track with your diet. I'll add in the nutritional value whenever possible, although I don't have those exact numbers for every recipe.

Easy Cobb Salad (Serves 1)

Ingredients:

1 cup of Spinach

2 strips of Bacon

1 Hard Boiled Egg

2 ounces of Chicken Breast

1/4 of an Avocado

1/2 of a Campari Tomato

1 tablespoon of Olive Oil

1/2 teaspoon of White Vinegar

Directions:

1. Cook chicken and bacon if not cooked yet.

2. Chop ingredients up into bite sized pieces.

3. Combine all ingredients in large bowl and add vinegar and oil.

4. Toss well.

5. Serve and Enjoy!

Nutritional Value:

43 grams of Protein.

48 grams of Fat.

3 grams of Carbs.

600 Calories.

Caprese Salad (Serves 2)

Ingredients:

1 large Tomato

1/2 pound of Fresh Mozzarella

1 tablespoon of Olive Oil

1 tablespoon of Balsamic Reduction

4 Basil Leaves

1 pinch of Pepper

1 pinch of Salt

Directions:

1. Wash then cut tomato into 1 centimeter sized slices.

2. Do the same thing with Mozzarella.

3. Arrange ingredients on a plate in alternating pattern.

4. Add some pepper and salt.

5. Drizzle olive oil and balsamic reduction on top.

6. Place basil leaves on top.

7. Serve and Enjoy!

Nutritional Value - (Serving Size 1/2 of Salad):

9 grams of Protein.

12 grams of Fat.

9 grams of Carbs.

189 Calories.

Simple Taco Salad (Serves 6)

Ingredients:

32 ounces of Ground Pork

9 ounces of Shredded Cheddar Cheese

6 teaspoons of McCormick Taco Seasoning

12 tablespoons of Salsa

12 tablespoons of Sour Cream

Cayenne Pepper

6 Romaine Leafs

Directions:

1. Brown your pork in skillet.

2. Add spices and taco seasoning once meat is browned.

3. Cook until taco seasoning is incorporated.

4. Allow to cool and evenly divide into 6 containers.

5. Add cheese to each of the containers.

6. Add Romaine to containers.

7. Add salsa and sour cream to your bowl.

8. Serve and Enjoy!

Nutritional Value - (Serving Size 1/6):

38 grams of Protein.

51 grams of Fat.

5 grams of Carbs.

647 Calories.

Grilled Halloumi Salad (Serves 1)

Ingredients:

1 Persian Cucumber

3 ounces of Halloumi Cheese

5 Grape Tomatoes

1/2 ounce of Chopped Walnuts

1 handful of Baby Arugula

Balsamic Vinegar

Olive Oil

Salt

Directions:

1. Cut your halloumi cheese into approximately 1/3 inch sized slices.

2. Grill these slices for 3 to 5 minutes on both sides. Should have nice grill marks on both sides.

3. Prep your salad by washing then cutting your vegetables. Tomatoes in half and cucumbers into smaller slices. Chop your walnuts and add them in your salad bowl.

4. Wash baby arugula and add to your bowl.

5. Arrange grilled halloumi cheese on top of salad. Add some salt. Dress salad with balsamic vinegar and olive oil.

6. Serve and Enjoy!

Nutritional Value:

21 grams of Protein.

47 grams of Fat.

7 grams of Carbs.

560 Calories.

Berry & Chicken Summer Salad (Serves 2)

Ingredients:

1 Chicken Breast

6 Diced Strawberries

2 cups of Spinach

3/4 cup of Blueberries

3 tablespoons of Crumbled Feta Cheese

3 tablespoons of Raspberry Balsamic Vinegar

1/2 cup of Chopped Walnuts

Directions:

1. Cut chicken breast up into small cubes and cook in your pan. When done place on your plate to cool off.

2. Gather your other ingredients and add them to a big bowl. Add your dressing.

3. Add your chicken and toss the salad.

4. Serve and Enjoy!

Nutritional Value:

21 grams of Protein.

19 grams of Fat.

16 grams of Carbs.

335 Calories.

Simple Chicken Salad (Serves 6)

Ingredients:

4 Chicken Breasts

105 grams of Green Peppers

125 grams of Celery

20 grams of Green Onions

3/4 Cup of Mayo

3/4 Cup of Sugar-Free Sweet Relish

3 Large Hardboiled Eggs

Directions:

1. Preheat your oven to 350 degrees.

2. Add your chicken to your oven safe pan.

3. Cook for approximately 45 to 60 minutes until your chicken is finished cooking.

4. Place 3 eggs in your pan and cover them with water. Bring it to a boil and then cook approximately 15 minutes once water is boiling.

5. While chicken is in oven cooking, chop up your onions, celery, and peppers.

6. Once your chicken is out of your oven let it cool down and then chop up.

7. Combine all ingredients in a large bowl.

8. Chop up your eggs and mix in. Add eggs last.

9. Split into 6 separate portions or containers.

10. Serve and Enjoy!

Nutritional Value - (Serving Size 1/6):

43 grams of Protein.

25 grams of Fat.

2 grams of Carbs.

413 Calories.

Easy Buffalo Wings (Serves 2)

Ingredients:

6 Chicken Wings (6 Drumettes & 6 Wingettes)

2 tablespoons of Butter

1/2 cup of Frank's Red Hot Sauce

Paprika

Garlic Powder

Pepper

Salt

Cayenne (optional)

Directions:

1. Break each chicken wing into 2 different pieces. The drumettes and wingettes, getting rid of the tips.

2. Pour hot sauce over your wings. Enough to lightly coat them.

3. Season wings with spices and cover them. Place in refrigerator for 1 hour.

4. Place broiler on high and put your oven rack 6 inches from broiler. Put your aluminum paper on a baking sheet. Place wings on your sheet with enough room so the flames can reach their sides.

5. Cook for 8 minutes under your broiler. Wings should turn dark brown on top. May turn black if very close to the flame.

6. Melt your butter on the oven top and add rest of hot sauce. Can also add cayenne if you want wings to be spicier.

7. Once butter has melted take off heat.

8. Take wings from broiler and flip them. Cook another 6 to 8 minutes.

9. Once good and browned on all sides take out of your broiler and add to bowl.

10. Pour butter-hot sauce mixture over wings. Toss wings to coat evenly.

11. Serve and Enjoy!

Nutritional Value - (Serving Size 6 Wings):

48 grams of Protein.

46 grams of Fat.

1 gram of Carbs:

620 Calories.

Oopsie Rolls (Serves 12)

Ingredients:

3 Large Eggs

1/8 teaspoon of Cream of Tartar

3 ounces of Cream Cheese

1/8 teaspoon of Salt

Directions:

1. Preheat your oven to 300 degrees.

2. Separate eggs from egg yolks. Place each in different bowls.

3. With an electric hand mixer beat your egg whites until they get very bubbly.

4. Add in your cream of tarter. Beat it until a stiff peak is formed.

5. In egg yolk bowl, add your 3 ounces of cream cheese and salt.

4. Beat egg yolk mixture until your yolks are a pale looking yellow and they have doubled in their size.

5. Fold the egg whites into the egg yolk mixture. Don't use an electric hand mixer. Gently fold it together.

6. Line a cookie sheet with parchment paper and spray with some oil or grease. Dollop your batter as big as you want them. I make 12 of equal size and the nutritional value amount reflects that.

7. Bake approximately 30 to 40 minutes. They are done when the tops of oopsie rolls are firm and golden.

8. Let cool on wire rack.

9. Serve and Enjoy!

<u>Nutritional Value - (Serving Size 1 Roll):</u>

2.3 grams of Protein

3.8 grams of Fat.

0 grams of Carbs.

45 Calories

Cucumber Sushi Rolls (Serves 2)

Ingredients:

1/2 pound of Tuna Steak

2 Cucumbers

1/2 of an Avocado

8 Shrimp

2 tablespoons of Mayonnaise

2 teaspoons of Sriracha

1/2 teaspoon of Sesame Seeds

1 stalk of Green Onion

Directions:

1. Peel your cucumbers and cut off their ends. You want to have two 6 to 8 inch long cylindrical shaped cucumbers when done.

2. Use a wet long knife and lay the edge of it against an edge of your cucumber. Begin cutting into it. Knife should be barely visible under your transparent cucumber.

3. Once cucumber is cut to its seeds gather your other ingredients.

4. Mix mayo and sriracha to make spicy mayo.

5. You're now ready to begin rolling! Take the end of your cucumber with your fish and begin rolling it onto itself. Make sure to keep your roll tight so that no air pockets form. The ingredients need to stick to one another, otherwise, they'll fall right out.

6. Once you're almost done rolling it and only have approximately 2 to 3 inches left of your cucumber, spread some of your spicy mayo on your cucumber and finish the roll. The mayonnaise will act as sort of glue to help keep your cucumber sealed.

7. Next, carefully slice your cucumber into 1/2 inch to 1-inch rounds. Hold both sides of your cucumber as slicing to help maintain its shape.

8. You should now have 6 to 8 pieces of sushi per roll. Chop up green onion and sprinkle on top.

9. Serve and Enjoy!

Nutritional Value:

36 grams of Protein.

17 grams of Fat.

2.5 grams of Carbs.

322 Calories.

Tuna Tartare (Serves 2)

Ingredients:

1 pound of Tuna Steak

3 stalks of Scallion

1 Avocado

1 tablespoon of Soy Sauce

2 tablespoons of Olive Oil

2 tablespoons of Sesame Seed Oil

1 teaspoon of Jalapeno

1 tablespoon of Mayo

1 tablespoon of Sriracha

1 tablespoon of Soy Sauce

1 teaspoon of Sesame Seeds

1/2 of a Lime

2 Persian Cucumbers

Directions:

1. Dice your tuna steak and your avocado into 1/4 inch cubes. Put them in your bowl.

2. Dice your jalapeno and scallion. Add them to bowl.

3. Pour sesame oil, olive oil, soy sauce, mayo, juice from a lime, and sriracha into your bowl.

4. Gently combine your ingredients using your hands.

5. Slice your Persian cucumber and sprinkle with sesame seeds.

6. Serve and Enjoy!

Nutritional Value:

56.75 grams of Protein.

24.5 grams of Fat.

4 grams of Carbs

487 Calories.

Simple Cucumber Sandwich (Serves 1)

Ingredients:

1 Cucumber

Sliced Meat

1.5 ounces of Boursin Cheese

Directions:

1. Slice your cucumber into half and use your melon baller to remove any seeds and some of the cucumber itself.

2. Fill the one side with a spreadable Boursin cheese.

3. Fold your sliced deli meat longways so you can fill the other half.

4. Serve and Enjoy!

Nutritional Value: (Will Vary on Type of Deli Meat Used)

17 grams of Protein.

12 grams of Fat.

7 grams of Carbs.

196 Calories.

Easy Tomato Soup (Serves 4)

Ingredients:

1 quart of Tomato Soup

4 tablespoons of Butter

1/4 cup of Olive Oil

1/4 cup of Frank's Red Hot Sauce

2 tablespoons of Apple Cider Vinegar

Spices

2 teaspoons of Black Pepper

1 tablespoon of Pink Himalayan Sea Salt

2 teaspoons of Turmeric

1 teaspoon of Oregano

Toppings

8 strips of Bacon

4 tablespoons of Creme Fraiche

Green Onion

Fresh Basil

Directions:

1. Cook bacon on your pan until it is crisp. Prepare tomato soup.

2. Combine all main ingredients in your pot. Set to a medium heat and stir.

3. Add in your spices.

4. Cook until butter is melted. Don't allow soup to boil. You want it to get to a nice simmer.

5. Pour into your soup bowls and top with creme fraiche, green onion, basil, and bacon.

6. Serve and Enjoy!

Nutritional Value - (Serving Size 1/4 of Soup):

11 grams of Protein.

37.5 grams of Fat.

16 grams of Carbs.

460 Calories.

Cheddar Broccoli Soup (Serves 4)

Ingredients:

1/2 of a White Onion

1 tablespoon of Butter

1 cup of Heavy Cream

2 cups of Broth

2 cups of Water

8 ounces of Cheddar

12 ounces of Broccoli

1/2 teaspoon of Paprika

1/4 teaspoon of Xanthan Gum

Pepper

Salt

Directions:

1. Heat large size soup pot and add a tablespoon of butter.

2. Saute your garlic and onion till fragrant and your onion looks translucent.

3. Add broth, cream, and water. Let come to boil. Season with salt, paprika, and pepper.

4. While boiling rip your broccoli into florets and measure 12 ounces. Place into boiling soup broth and reduce it to a simmer. Allow your broccoli to cook for approximately 25 minutes.

5. Once broccoli is cooked, add in 8 ounces of cheddar cheese and stir it in till melted. I prefer cubed cheese but shredded works better as it melts quicker.

6. After your cheese has melted, turn the heat off. Pour the contents into a large blender and continue to blend till contents are smooth. You can also use an immersion blender if you prefer.

7. When blending, slowly add in a 1/4 teaspoon of your xanthan gum. You should notice your soup thickening.

8. When finished, sprinkle some cheddar cheese on top.

9. Serve and Enjoy!

Nutritional Value - (Serving Size 1.5 Cups):

11 grams of Protein.

32 grams of Fat.

8 grams of Carbs.

370 Calories.

Avgolemono Soup (Serves 8)

Ingredients:

3 Eggs

2 tablespoons of Olive Oil

1 medium Onion

6 cups of Chicken Broth

4 Shredded Chicken Breasts

1/2 cup of Heavy Cream

2 cups of Water

2 Juiced Lemons

1/2 head of Riced Cauliflower

Chopped Parsley

Dill

Pepper

Salt

Directions:

1. Rice your head of cauliflower by removing leaves and chopping into large sized florets. Grate your florets on coarsest side of your box grater a few times.

2. Cook chicken in an oiled pan. Once cooked pull the meat apart until it is in small pieces.

3. In a big oiled pot cook your onions over medium heat until turning brown and translucent.

4. Add your water, chicken broth, heavy cream, riced cauliflower, and chicken.

5. Add in your herbs and lemon juice. Taste and make sure your soup has lemon flavor and is salted enough to your liking.

6. Cook for approximately 8 minutes until your cauliflower gets tender.

7. While your soup is cooking get a bowl and beat together your eggs in it. While whisking the eggs with your one hand, pour a ladle of your soup broth into the eggs with your other hand slowly so it doesn't cook the eggs unevenly.

8. When eggs have 1 to 2 ladles full of the soup broth in them turn flame under your pot off.

9. Pour egg mixture into soup slowly, stirring your soup while pouring.

10. Don't turn the heat back on. Let the soup bring your eggs to their full temp for approximately 2 to 3 minutes.

11. Add some pepper and chopped parsley.

12. Serve and Enjoy!

Nutritional Value - (Serving Size 1/8 of Soup):

20.7 grams of Protein.

16.3 grams of Fat.

5.3 grams of Carbs.

251 Calories.

Buffalo Chicken Soup (Serves 4)

Ingredients:

4 Chicken Breasts

2 Carrots

4 stalks of Celery

6 tablespoons of Butter

2 ounces of Cream Cheese

1 quart of Chicken Broth

1/2 cup of Frank's Red Hot Sauce

1/2 cup of Heavy Cream

1/2 teaspoon of Cayenne

1/2 teaspoon of Thyme

1 teaspoon of Salt

Directions:

1 Set your celery and carrot to cook in your oiled pot.

2. When they've begun to break down put in your chicken breast to cook with them. Cover your pot to let them steam and cook faster.

3. Once your chicken is fully cooked remove from pot. By cooking your chicken this way it lets a slight crust begin to form around it that boiling wouldn't be able to achieve. Once it's cooked shred your chicken.

4. Pour your chicken broth over vegetables. Add in cream cheese, heavy cream, and butter.

5. While that's coming to a boil place your now shredded chicken back into the soup.

6. Add hot sauce.

7. Add all herbs. Let your soup simmer for around 15 to 20 minutes. This will allow your flavors to marry.

8. Garnish your soup however you'd like. I use green onion and cold sour cream.

9. Serve and Enjoy!

Nutritional Value - (Serving Size 1/4 of Soup):

57 grams of Protein.

32.5 grams of Fat.

4 grams of Carbs.

563 Calories.

Seafood Soup (Serves 6)

Ingredients:

<u>Soup</u>

8 ounces of Calamari

10 ounces of Wild Caught Cod

8 ounces of Shrimp

1 1/2 cups of Tomato Sauce

1/3 cup of Coconut Oil

1/2 cup of Coconut Cream

1 quart of Seafood Broth

3 medium Carrots

2 cups of Water

4 stalks of Green Onion

4 stalks of Celery

1 medium Onion

4 cloves of Garlic

8 ounces of Mushrooms

1 Lemon

1 Lime

Spices

2 teaspoons of Pepper

1 tablespoon of Salt

2 teaspoons of Red Pepper Flakes

1 teaspoon of Thyme

1 teaspoon of Dill

2 teaspoons of Basil

2 teaspoons of Oregano

3 Whole Bay Leaves

Fresh Parsley

Directions:

1. Start with 2 tablespoons of coconut oil in your soup pot over a medium flame.

2. Throw in your crushed garlic and onions. Cook them until they are fragrant.

3. Throw in your chopped celery and carrots. Let cook until they are tender.

4. Pour in 1 quart of broth, tomato sauce, and water.

5. Let come to boil. Reduce heat to a simmer. Let vegetables and broth simmer approximately 30 minutes. Season at this time.

6. While soup is still simmering, peel your shrimp. Set to the side.

7. Cut calamari tubes into 1/2 inch pieces and set them in your bowl with lemon juice.

8. Chop mushrooms up and add to soup after the soup has been simmering for 30 minutes. Add your coconut cream. Make sure soup returns to simmer if your cream cooled off the soup too much.

9. Once mushrooms have cooked for approximately 10 minutes add in your cod and cook for another 10 minutes.

10. Break fish down in your pot using your wooden spoon to break it into smaller pieces.

11. Make sure water is simmering before cooking shrimp. Turn the heat up a little bit and add shrimp. Cook approximately 3 minutes.

12. After 3 minutes add in your calamari to the soup. Don't add in lemon juice. Let cook for 2 more minutes. Any longer and calamari may get rubbery and the shrimp might start getting hard.

13. Take pot off the heat. Add in lime juice. Top with fresh parsley and chopped green onion. Remove the bay leaves.

14. Serve and Enjoy!

Nutritional Value - (Serving Size 1/6 of Soup):

27 grams of Protein.

14 grams of Fat.

9 grams of Carbs.

284 Calories.

Chili Chicken Soup (Serves 8)

Ingredients:

8 Boneless Chicken Thighs

1 Pepper

1 Onion

8 slices of Bacon

2 tablespoons of Unsalted Butter

1 tablespoon of Thyme

1 tablespoon of Coconut Flour

1 tablespoon of Minced Garlic

3 tablespoons of Lemon Juice

1 teaspoon of Pepper

1 teaspoon of Salt

1 cup of Chicken Stock

3 tablespoons of Tomato Paste

1/4 cup of Unsweetened Coconut Milk

Directions:

1. Put a pat of butter in the center of your crockpot.

2. Slice peppers and onions thinly. Distribute them evenly over bottom of crockpot.

3. Cover them with your boneless chicken thighs.

4. Cut up your bacon and place over chicken.

5. Add your coconut flour, pepper, salt, and garlic.

6. Add your liquids (chicken stock, lemon juice, and coconut milk).

7. Add tomato paste.

8. Cook on low approximately 6 hours.

9. Stir and break up your chicken before you serve.

10. Serve and Enjoy!

Nutritional Value - (Serving Size 1/8 of Soup):

41 grams of Protein.

21 grams of Fat.

7 grams of Carbs.

396 Calories.

Spicy Tomato Basil Soup (Serves 6)

Ingredients:

3 pounds of Plum Tomatoes

6 cloves of Garlic

1 Sweet Onion

3 tablespoons of Olive Oil

2 tablespoons of Butter

1 quart of Broth

1/2 cup of Basil

2 tablespoons of Tomato Paste

Spices

1/2 teaspoon of Pepper

1 tablespoon of Salt

1/2 teaspoon of Thyme

1 tablespoon of Sriracha

1/2 teaspoon of Paprika

1 teaspoon of Crushed Red Pepper

1/2 teaspoon of Cayenne

Directions:

1. Divide your tomatoes into thirds. 1/3 will be saved as fresh tomato and the other 2/3 will be roasted.

2. Wash and dry 8 plum tomatoes. Cut in half lengthwise and lay out on a cookie sheet that has been greased, cut side up. Sprinkle these tomatoes with salt and olive oil and bake them in the oven for approximately 40 minutes at 400 degrees. You'll notice the tomatoes get wrinkled and darker as moisture leaves them.

3. While tomatoes roast, cut up a sweet onion and squeeze your garlic through your garlic press. Add in a tablespoon of olive oil to a big soup pot and cook your garlic and onion until they are translucent and fragrant.

4. Cut fresh tomatoes into small pieces and throw them into garlic and onion. Pour broth into the pot and let it come to a boil.

5. Add your basil leaves. Make sure they've been chopped up first. Add some butter and tomato paste to the pot.

6. Add your spices. Make it as hot or spicy as you prefer.

7. Boil your spicy mixture over a medium heat while tomatoes are roasting.

8. Once tomatoes are finished roasting, take them out and add them into your spicy mixture. Lower the heat to low and allow to simmer for approximately 40 minutes.

9. Ladle a good portion of your soup into your blender or Nutribullet. Blend for a few seconds. The longer you do this the creamier it will get. Don't blend too long. If using a Nutribullet open your blending cap slowly so steam is released slowly. If you do it too fast hot soup could shoot out and lead to burns.

10. Top with green onion, sour cream, or shredded cheese. Whatever you prefer.

11. Serve and Enjoy!

Nutritional Value - (Serving Size 1/6 of Soup):

3 grams of Protein.

12 grams of Fat.

9 grams of Carbs.

164 Calories.

Bacon Cheddar Cauliflower Soup (Serves 6)

Ingredients:

4 slices of Bacon

1 Cauliflower Head

1 medium Onion

2 tablespoons of Olive Oil

1 teaspoon of Ground Thyme

12 ounces of Aged Cheddar

3 cups of Chicken Broth

1/4 cup of Heavy Cream

1 tablespoon of Minced Garlic

1 ounce of Parmesan Cheese

Directions:

1. Dice your cauliflower and place on your foil lined baking sheet. Drizzle it with your olive oil.

2. Separately pepper and salt your cauliflower and bacon. Cook cauliflower for 35 minutes at 375 degrees.

3. Cook your bacon until it is crisp.

4. Ideally using a large pot that will fit your soup, dice your medium onion and fry it up in your bacon grease.

5. Once onion is cooked, add thyme and garlic and cook for between 30 seconds and 1 minute.

6. Add your cauliflower and chicken broth. Simmer while covered for approximately 20 minutes.

7. While cauliflower simmers, shred your aged cheddar.

8. Using your immersion blender, blend cauliflower into your soup.

9. Add cheese and blend some more.

10. Add cream and bacon. Mix together with a spoon.

11. Serve and Enjoy!

Nutritional Value - (Serving Size 1/6):

18 grams of Protein.

25 grams of Fat.

11 grams of Carbs.

337 Calories.

Easy Lobster Bisque (Serves 4)

Ingredients:

24 ounces of Lobster Chunks

1/2 of Red Onion

4 cloves of Garlic

2 Carrots

1/2 cup of Tomato Paste

4 stalks of Celery

1 quart of Seafood Broth

1 tablespoon of Olive Oil

2 cups of White Wine

1 ounce of Brandy

3 Bay Leaves

1 cup of Heavy Cream

1 teaspoon of Peppercorns

1 tablespoon of Salt

1 teaspoon of Thyme

1 teaspoon of Paprika

1 tablespoon of Fresh Lemon Juice

1 teaspoon of Xanthan Gum

Parsley

Directions:

1. Chop garlic, carrots, celery, and onion.

2. In a soup pot cook your onion in olive oil until fragrant. Add garlic and cook till pan starts looking black and crusty at the bottom.

3. Deglaze your pot using white wine. Add your carrot and celery.

4. Pour in broth, tomato paste, and brandy. Stir to help incorporate.

5. Add spices and let your soup simmer for 60 minutes.

6. Once soup is cooked remove and discard your bay leaves.

7. Add your cream and allow soup to come to a simmer.

8. Add in small portion xanthan gum slowly while stirring your soup. Should see soup thicken.

9. Pour soup into your blender. Blend soup before adding lobster chunks. If you want chunkier bisque don't blend at all. If blending continue to do so until it is creamy.

10. If lobster isn't cooked, cut into chunks and saute in some olive oil and butter in a pan.

11. Pour bisque into bowl and add your lobster chunks. Stir well until it is combined.

12. Dress your bisque with some green onion, lemon juice, and parsley.

13. Serve and Enjoy!

Nutritional Value - (Serving Size 1/4 of Bisque):

12 grams of Protein.

15 grams of Fat.

8 grams of Carbs.

220 Calories.

Simple Clam Chowder (Serves 4)

Ingredients:

3 strips of Bacon

1 Carrot

1 Onion

2 tablespoons of Butter

2 stalks of Celery

4 cloves of Garlic

1 cup of Clam Juice

2 1/2 cups of Heavy Cream

1 cup of Water

1 teaspoon of Xanthan Gum

1/2 a head of Cauliflower

16 ounces of Canned Clams

1 teaspoon of Parsley

1 teaspoon of Pepper

1 teaspoon of Salt

1/2 teaspoon of Celery Salt

1/2 teaspoon of Thyme

Directions:

1. Set your pot of water to boil.

2. Cut half a head of your cauliflower into medium size florets. Throw cauliflower into the water once boiling and cook for 10 minutes. They should get very soft by the time they're done.

3. While cauliflower boils, chop your other ingredients. Bacon should be in 1/2 inch cubed pieces. Carrot and onion should be minced. Celery should be cut into slices that are a 1/4 inch.

4. Throw your bacon in a large soup pot on medium heat and cook until it is crispy. Once bacon is cooked, add in onion, celery, and carrot. Sprinkle with a little salt and cook until your onion begins to turn translucent.

5. Add in some butter and squeezed garlic.

6. Open canned clams and separate juice by putting your strainer in a bowl and pouring canned clams in. Save both juice and the clams.

7. By now your cauliflower should be done. Drain water and put them into your blender or a Nutribullet with a bit of water. Blend them until they are creamy.

8. Add your blended cauliflower, water, clam juice, heavy cream, and vegetables to the bacon. Lower flame to low heat and allow to simmer for approximately 20 minutes.

9. Spice chowder with celery salt, pepper, salt. Add thyme last.

10. Add in xanthan gum.

11. Add clams. Cook clams till warmed up. Should be 5 minutes at the most. Overcooking the clams will leave them tough and very chewy.

12. Sprinkle some thyme on top of chowder.

13. Serve and Enjoy!

<u>Nutritional Value - (Serving Size 1/4 of Chowder):</u>

28 grams of Protein.

66 grams of Fat.

15 grams of Carbs.

804 Calories.

Easy Beef Stew (Serves 6)

Ingredients:

5 pounds of Beef Shank

3 medium Carrots

2 medium Onions

8 Campari Tomatoes

8 cloves of Garlic

2 cups of Water

1 quart of Chicken Broth

2 tablespoons of Apple Cider Vinegar

1/4 cup of Tomato Sauce

Spices

3 teaspoons of Crushed Red Pepper

4 teaspoons of Salt

2 teaspoons of Basil

3 Whole Bay Leaves

2 teaspoons of Onion Powder

2 teaspoons of Parsley

2 teaspoons of Black Pepper

2 teaspoons of Garlic Powder

1 teaspoon of Cayenne

Directions:

1. Place your cast iron skill on medium heat while you chop tomatoes, onion, carrots, and garlic into chunky sized pieces.

2. Place your garlic, carrots, and onions into a soup pot that's been oiled or a Dutch oven. Cook until onions are translucent.

3. In your hot cast iron skillet sear each side of all your beef shanks till a deep brown crust has formed. You're not cooking the beef now, just letting it develop a nice crust that you couldn't get by boiling.

4. Pour chicken broth over your carrots, onions, and garlic. Add water and apple cider vinegar.

5. Add your tomatoes, spices, and tomato sauce. Stir it well.

6. When beef shanks are seared, submerge them each into your broth and allow it to boil.

7. After your stew has come to boil, reduce your heat to a simmer. Let simmer uncovered slightly for approximately 3 hours. Cook until meat is completely cooked and tender.

8. Remove the bay leaves.

9. Serve and Enjoy!

Nutritional Value - (Serving Size 1/6 of Stew):

68 grams of Protein.

22 grams of Fat.

9 grams of Carbs.

531 Calories.

Roasted Brussels Sprouts w/ Bacon (Serves 4)

Ingredients:

8 strips of Bacon

1 pound of Brussels Sprouts

2 tablespoons of Olive Oil.

Pepper

Salt

Directions:

1. Preheat your oven to 375 degrees. Cut off ends of each of your Brussels sprouts. Then cut them down into halves.

2. Put in a large bowl and mix with salt, pepper, olive oil, and other spice you prefer to use. Sometimes I add red pepper.

3. Pour out onto a greased baking sheet. Leave some room between them.

4. Bake in your oven for approximately 30 minutes. About halfway in, grab your sheet in the oven and give a strong shake so that they rotate a bit.

5. Fry up your bacon while Brussels sprouts are cooking. I do two slices per serving.

6. Once bacon is cooked, chop it into small pieces about 1/2 inch big.

7. Once Brussels sprouts have blackened and shriveled a little they are ready. Take out of your oven and put into a bowl with your bacon. Toss it together and sprinkle some salt on top.

8. Serve and Enjoy!

Nutritional Value:

15 grams of Protein.

21 grams of Fat.

4 grams of Carbs.

278 Calories.

Bacon Wrapped Jalapeno Poppers (Serves 4)

Ingredients:

16 strips of Bacon

16 Fresh Jalapenos

4 ounces of Cream Cheese

1 teaspoon of Salt

1/4 cup of Shredded Cheddar Cheese

1 teaspoon of Paprika

Directions:

1. Preheat your oven to 350 degrees.

2. Slice pieces of bacon in half.

3. Slice ends off the jalapenos. Slice each one lengthwise in half. Remove membranes and seeds with knife or corer. I suggest wearing gloves to protect your hands.

4. Mix cheddar cheese and cream cheese together in a bowl.

5. Fill each half of your jalapenos with this cheese mixture.

6. Wrap your jalapenos in bacon.

7. Place these bacon wrapped jalapenos on a baking sheet that is lined with aluminum foil. Leave some room between each jalapeno.

8. Bake for approximately 20 to 25 minutes.

9. Add your paprika, salt, and any other desired spices.

10. Serve and Enjoy!

<u>Nutritional Value - (Serving Size 4 Jalapenos):</u>

10.2 grams of Protein.

17.9 grams of Fat.

3.3 grams of Carbs.

225 Calories.

Bacon Cheesy Wrapped Hot Dogs (Serves 4)

Ingredients:

8 strips of Bacon

8 Sausage Links

16 slices of Pepper Jack Cheese

Onion Powder

Garlic Powder

Black Pepper

Paprika

Toothpicks

Directions:

1. Preheat your oven to 400 degrees.

2. Cook your sausage links on a grill or oiled pan until nearly done. Take off heat and allow to cool until you can handle them.

3. Cut slits in the middle of each one until they are butterflied. The deeper the cut, the more cheese will fit.

4. Take 2 slices of your cheese and place into the middle of each of your sausage links.

5. Tightly wrap each link in bacon. Secure it with a wet toothpick.

6. Sprinkle on your spices and bake until your bacon gets crispy. Should take approximately 15 to 20 minutes. I suggest flipping them halfway through.

7. Remove from oven.

8. Serve and Enjoy!

<u>Nutritional Value - (Serving Size 2 Hot Dogs):</u>

40 grams of Protein.

41 grams of Fat.

4 grams of Carbs.

570 Calories.

Spicy & Sweet Chicken & Shrimp (Serves 2)

Ingredients:

20 Large Shrimped (De-Veined and Peeled)

2 Boneless Chicken Breasts

2 handfuls of Spinach

1/2 pound of Mushrooms

2 tablespoons of Sriracha

1/4 cup of Mayo

2 teaspoons of Lime Juice

1 tablespoon of Coconut Oil

1 teaspoon of Garlic Powder

1 teaspoon of Salt

1/2 teaspoon of Erythritol

1/2 teaspoon of Paprika

1/2 teaspoon of Crushed Red Pepper

1 stalk of Green Onion

1/4 teaspoon of Xanthan Gum

Directions:

1. Tenderize chicken breasts.

2. Place chicken breast on an oiled large pan and cook over medium-high heat. Season them with garlic powder and salt. Cook for approximately 8 minutes before flipping. Reduce your heat and cover it when flipped onto its other side.

3. Slice mushrooms and throw them into pan around your chicken as it's cooking. Season them garlic powder and salt. Add more oil if necessary.

4. In a separate pan, we'll cook your shrimp and sauce. Get shrimp ready for cooking. Make sure shrimp are peeled and deveined.

5. Combine sriracha, mayo, xanthan gum, and erythritol. Whisk quickly and well.

6. Heat your pan over medium heat. Lay out shrimp in an even layer. Quickly combine shrimp and sauce. Toss completely to coat each of your shrimp. Cook for approximately 3 minutes while stirring often.

7. Once shrimp are done, turn off heat and remove pan. Add your lime juice and toss them again.

8. Prepare a spinach bed and add your cooked mushrooms on top of it.

9. Place chicken on top of spinach bed and top it with as much shrimp as you want.

10. Garnish with your green onion and some lime wedges.

Nutritional Value:

50 grams of Protein.

39 grams of Fat.

3 grams of Carbs.

591 Calories.

Coconut Shrimp (Serves 2)

Ingredients:

Shrimp

12 Large Shrimp

15 grams of Flaked Coconut

30 grams of Shredded Coconut

1 Egg Yolk

3 tablespoons of Unsweetened Coconut Milk

6 tablespoons of Mayo

Dip

4 tablespoons of Mayonnaise

1 teaspoon of Unsweetened Lime Juice

2 teaspoons of Chili Garlic Sauce

Directions:

1. Thaw out and dry your shrimp.

2. Mix the rest of shrimp ingredients together.

3. Coat your shrimp in this mixture.

4. Drop your shrimp into the fryer and cook until they are golden brown.

5. Mix together all your dip ingredients.

6. Serve and Enjoy!

Nutritional Value - (Serving Size 6 Shrimp):

11 grams of Protein.

69 grams of Fat.

7 grams of Carbs.

670 Calories.

Brussels Sprouts Burgers (Serves 14)

Ingredients:

32 ounces of Brussels Sprouts

36 grams of Green Onion

3 Eggs

1/3 cup of Almond Flour

8 ounces of Parmesan Cheese

11 ounces of Goat Cheese

Pepper

Salt

Directions:

1. Wash your Brussels sprouts and shred them using the grater setting on your food processor.

2. Finely grate your Parmesan cheese and mix with your Brussels sprouts, almond flour, pepper, and salt.

3. Crumble your goat cheese into mixture and combine with your hands.

4. Beat the 3 eggs together and combine with rest of mixture.

5. Patty out 4 ounces Brussels Sprouts burgers.

6. Heat your oil in a cast iron skillet.

7. Fry your burgers for 2 1/2 minutes on each side until crisp.

8. Serve and Enjoy!

<u>Nutritional Value - (Serving Size 1/14):</u>

14 grams of Protein.

11 grams of Fat.

7 grams of Carbs.

182 Calories.

Keto Quarter Pounder (Serves 2)

Ingredients:

1/2 pound of Ground Beef

1 strip of Bacon

1 Egg

1 tablespoon of Mayo

1 tablespoon of Sliced Pickled Jalapenos

1/4 of an Onion

1/2 of a Plum Tomato

1 tablespoon of Sriracha

2 Leaves of Lettuce

2 tablespoons of Butter

Spices

1/2 teaspoon of Crushed Red Pepper

1/2 teaspoon of Salt

1/2 teaspoon of Basil

1/4 teaspoon of Cayenne

Directions:

1. Knead meat for 3 minutes.

2. Chop and dice ingredients finely.

3. Add your bacon, eggs, tomato, 1 tablespoon of butter, and spices together to meat and knead the meat again.

4. Split your meat in half two times and flatten all 4 pieces of meat to make flat-sized patties. Add a tablespoon of butter to the center of two pieces of meat and then put on the non-buttered pieces. Seal up their sides so you get 2 big patties that are ready for grilling.

5. Put patties on the grill. Throw onions on your grill after flipping burgers at the 5-minute mark.

6. Flip your onions after 2 1/2 minutes to cook evenly on both sides. Cook burger for additional 5 minutes. Total cook time for your burger is approximately 10 minutes.

7. Place your patties on two big leaves of lettuce and place on your mayo. Top with whatever toppings you prefer. I use sriracha and sliced jalapenos.

Nutritional Value - (Serving Size 1 Burger):

25 grams of Protein.

34 grams of Fat.

4 grams of Carbs.

443 Calories.

Sloppy Joe's (Serves 2)

Ingredients:

Meat

3 strips of Bacon (chopped)

1 pound of Ground Beef

3 Plum Tomatoes

1/2 cup of Chopped Onion

3 cloves of Garlic

1 teaspoon of Dark Brown Sugar

1/4 cup of Ketchup

1 teaspoon of Lemon Juice

2 tablespoons of Mustard

1/2 teaspoon of Soy Sauce

1/2 teaspoon of White Vinegar

2 tablespoons of Sriracha

Spices

1 dash of Cayenne

1 teaspoon of Salt

1 dash of Crushed Red Pepper

1 dash of Garlic Powder

1 dash of Thyme

1 dash of Basil

For Sandwich

2 Pretzel Buns

1 Sliced Jalapeno

1 tablespoon of Butter

1/2 cup of Shredded Pepper Jack

Directions:

1. Chop up bacon and onion. Throw bacon in your hot pan over medium heat and spread out so it all cooks the same. Once your bacon is browned and your pan is oiled up nicely with bacon grease, throw in your onion and cook until it is translucent.

2. Place a pot of water to boil. Just enough to cover two tomatoes. Once boiling, throw in tomatoes and boil for approximately 2 minutes. Take out of the water and allow to cool.

3. Remove tomato skins. Crush tomatoes in a pulp and then squeeze garlic into them.

4. Once your onions are translucent, add your ground beef and begin breaking it into smallish chunks. Lower the flame and allow to simmer so nothing gets overcooked.

5. Add in crushed tomato and stir well.

6. Add in spices, sugar, sriracha, mustard, ketchup, vinegar, soy sauce, and lemon juice. Stir it well and continue to let simmer.

7. Shred pepper jack cheese.

8. Cut pretzel buns in half. In a different pan, melt butter until it is browned. Place buns with their flat side down on the butter to soak it and get toasted.

9. Once Sloppy Joe mixture is cooked and thicker turn off your heat.

10. Sprinkle cheese on your bottom bun and add Sloppy Joe. Top with sliced jalapeno if you want.

11. Serve and Enjoy!

Nutritional Value - (Serving Size 1/2 of Sloppy Joe without any type of bun):

73 grams of Protein.

46 grams of Fat.

18 grams of Carbs.

817 Calories.

Avocado Fries (Serves 3)

Ingredients:

1 Egg

3 Avocados

1 1/2 cups of Sunflower Oil

1 1/2 cups of Almond Meal

1/2 teaspoon of Salt

1/4 teaspoon of Cayenne Pepper

Directions:

1. Break egg into your bowl and beat. In a different bowl, mix your almond meal with cayenne pepper and salt.

2. Slice avocados in half and remove seeds.

3. Peel skin off of every half.

4. Slice avocado vertically into 4 pieces.

5. Heat deep fryer to 350 degrees.

6. Coat each slice of your avocado in the egg mixture. Roll each coated slice in your almond meal mix.

7. Carefully place each slice into your deep fryer. Do this carefully.

8. Fry for approximately 45 seconds to 1 minute until it is light brown.

9. Quickly transfer to plate with paper towel on it to soak up your excess oil.

10. Mix some mayo and sriracha sauce.

11. Serve and Enjoy!

<u>Nutritional Value - (Serving Size 1/3 of Fries):</u>

17 grams of Protein.

51 grams of Fat.

8 grams of Carbs.

587 Calories

Portobello Mushroom Pizza (Serves 3)

Ingredients:

3 Portobello Mushrooms

3 slices of Tomato

Drizzle of Olive Oil

3 teaspoons of Pizza Seasoning

12 Pepperoni Slices

9 Spinach leafs

1.5 ounces of Mozzarella

1.5 ounces of Cheddar Cheese

1.5 ounces of Monterey Jack

Directions:

1. Preheat your convection oven to 450 degrees.

2. De-stem and wash your Portobello mushrooms.

3. Place your mushrooms with cap side down on your foiled lined sheet. Drizzle it with olive oil.

4. Sprinkle with some pizza seasoning.

5. Layer your spinach, then tomato, then cheese, and a round of seasoning.

6. Cook for approximately 6 minutes until cheese melts.

7. Add your pepperoni and cook till your pepperoni is crispy.

8. Serve and Enjoy!

Nutritional Value - (Serving Size 1 Pizza):

19 grams of Protein.

21 grams of Fat.

6 grams of Carbs.

276 Calories.

Low-Carb Keto Pizza (Serves 3)

Ingredients:

Crust

1 Egg

3 tablespoons of Coconut Flour

4 tablespoons of Almond Flour

1 1/4 cup of Shredded Mozzarella

1 teaspoon of Oregano

1/2 teaspoon of Fennel Seed

1 teaspoon of Salt

1/2 teaspoon of Garlic Powder

1 teaspoon of Crushed Red Pepper

Pizza Toppings

1/2 Cup of Pizza Sauce

3 tablespoons of Ricotta Cheese

6 ounces of Sliced Fresh Mozzarella

2 tablespoons of Sliced Jalapenos

Directions:

Pizza Crust

1. Preheat your oven to 400 degrees.

2. Melt your shredded cheese in a toaster oven or your microwave until it is malleable and soft.

3. Add spices.

4. Add your almond flour, eggs, and coconut flour to your melted cheese to combine. Be sure all your ingredients are combined well (heat 10 seconds again if needed).

5. Place your dough between two sheets of parchment paper and then roll into your preferred shape. I go with round shape.

6. Bake at 400 degrees approximately 12 to 15 minutes or until slightly golden.

Pizza Toppings

7. Evenly spread out your sauce over the crust. Get sauce as close to edges as you prefer!

8. Lay out your sliced mozzarella over top the sauce. Add small globs of ricotta all around. You want some in every slice.

9. Add any other desired toppings.

10. Bake your pizza for approximately 10 minutes at 400 degrees until mozzarella is fully melted.

11. Serve and Enjoy!

Nutritional Values - (Serving Size 2 Slices):

30 grams of Protein.

42 grams of Fat.

13 grams of Carbs.

578 Calories.

Almond Bun Pizza (Serves 4)

Ingredients:

2 Eggs

5 tablespoons of Butter

3/4 cup of Almond Meal

1 1/2 teaspoons of Splenda

1 1/2 teaspoons of Baking Powder

1/2 teaspoon of Oregano

1/2 teaspoon of Garlic Powder

1/4 teaspoon of Thyme

1/2 cup of Alfredo Sauce

4 ounces of Cheddar

2 ounces of Jarlsberg

Directions:

1. Combine your dry ingredients and mix them well.

2. Be sure eggs are warmed up placing them in some hot water before using.

3. Add your eggs to the dry ingredients.

4. Melt butter and add to your mixture.

5. Spray some Pam on a pizza pan and spread mixture on the pan.

6. Cook for 7 minutes at 350 degrees.

7. Add your Alfredo sauce to the pizza.

8. Add your cheese and any other desired toppings.

9. Broil it for approximately 2 minutes.

10. Serve and Enjoy!

<u>Nutritional Value - (Serving Size 2):</u>

16 grams of Protein.

43 grams of Fat.

6 grams of Carbs.

462 Calories.

Spaghetti Squash Lasagna (Serves 12)

Ingredients:

3 pounds of Ground Beef

2 large Cooked Spaghetti Squash (1.25 kg)

30 slices of Mozzarella Cheese

32 ounces of Whole Milk Ricotta Cheese

40 ounces of Rao's Marinara Sauce

Directions:

1. Preheat your oven to 375 degrees.

2. Split your spaghetti squash and place them face down in your big glass dish. Fill with water till meat portion of your squash has been covered.

3. Bake approximately 45 minutes.

4. While baking start also browning your meat.

5. Add your meat to a large size saucepan. Add your marinara sauce. Set this aside once hot and mixed together.

6. When spaghetti squash is finished cooking scrap meat of squash from spaghetti.

7. Assemble your lasagna in a large sized greased pan. First, start with a layer of spaghetti squash followed by meat sauce, mozzarella, ricotta and repeat from beginning till all ingredients are used up.

8. Bake approximately 35 minutes. The top layer of your cheese should have begun to brown.

9. Serve and Enjoy!

Nutritional Value - (Serving Size 1/12 of Lasagna):

43 grams of Protein.

59 grams of Fat.

15 grams of Carbs.

711 Calories.

Mushroom & Shrimp Zucchini Pasta (Serves 1)

Ingredients:

12 ounces of Peeled Shrimp

2 tablespoons of Olive Oil

2 tablespoons of Butter

1/2 pound of White Mushrooms

1 large Zucchini

Parmesan Cheese

1/2 cup of Marinara Sauce

Red Pepper Flakes

Oregano

Basil

Pepper

Salt

Directions:

1. Heat up 2 tablespoons of your olive oil over medium heat in a large pan. Slice mushrooms and fry until they've soaked most of the oil up.

2. Add 2 tablespoons of your butter and allow mushrooms to cook till they turn golden.

3. Add your shrimp and cook approximately 4 minutes on both sides.

4. While your shrimp are cooking begin making your zoodles using a spiralizer. Twist zucchini to the spiralizer until it begins to resemble noodles.

5. Once shrimp have cooked, toss in your zoodles and mix all together. Cook approximately 2 minutes.

6. Add your marinara sauce and season with red pepper flakes, pepper, salt, oregano, and basil.

7. Toss everything together and sprinkle some Parmesan cheese on top.

8. Serve and Enjoy!

Nutritional Value:

39 grams of Protein.

28 grams of Fat.

7.5 grams of Carbs.

440 Calories.

Spaghetti Squash w/ Meatballs (Serves 10)

Ingredients:

Beef Meatballs:

16 ounces of Ground Beef (80/20)

1/3 of a Green Pepper

1/3 of an Onion

1 tablespoon of Minced Garlic

1 tablespoon of Coconut Flour

1 Egg

2 ounces of Shredded Cheddar Cheese

Pepper

Salt

Pork Meatballs:

16 ounces of Ground Pork

1/3 of a Green Pepper

1/3 of an Onion

1 Egg

1 tablespoon of Minced Garlic

1 tablespoon of Almond Flour

2 ounces of Shredded Monterey Jack Cheese

Pepper

Salt

Chicken Meatballs:

16 ounces of Ground Chicken Thighs

1/3 of a Green Pepper

1/3 of an Onion

1 Egg

1 tablespoon of Minced Garlic

1 tablespoon of Ground Flax Meal

2 ounces of Shredded Jarlsberg Cheese

Pepper

Salt

Spaghetti:

1 kilogram of Spaghetti Squash (cooked and shredded)

24 ounces of Rao's Homemade Marinara Sauce

10 teaspoons of Parmesan Cheese

Directions:

1. Cut your spaghetti squash in two and scrape out inside.

2. Place it face down in your glass container. Add some water till it goes above your cut portion.

3. Cook for approximately 45 minutes at 375 degrees.

4. Dice your onions and pepper. Divide up into three separate parts.

5. Combine your beef, 1/3 of your onions and peppers, 1 egg, coconut flour, pepper, salt, garlic, and cheddar cheese.

6. Divide this up into 10 separate meatballs. Should be about 1.5 ounces each.

7. Place them on a baking sheet that's been lined with foil.

8. Combine your pork, 1/3 of your onions and peppers, 1 egg, almond flour, pepper, salt, garlic, and Monterey Jack cheese.

9. Divide this up into 10 separate meatballs. Should be about 1.5 ounces each.

10. Place them on a baking sheet that's been lined with foil.

11. Combine your pork, 1/3 of your onions and peppers, 1 egg, ground flax meal, pepper, salt, garlic, and Jarlsberg cheese.

12. Divide this up into 10 separate meatballs. Should be about 1.5 ounces each.

13. Place them on a baking sheet that's been lined with foil.

14. Cook them at 375 degrees for approximately 25 minutes.

15. Using 10 containers - 1 per serving. Place 100 grams of spaghetti squash, 1 of each type of meatball, 2 ounces of marinara, and 1 ounce of shredded Parmesan cheese into each container.

<u>Nutritional Value - (Serving Size 3 Meatballs & 100 grams of Spaghetti Squash):</u>

45 grams of Protein.

21 grams of Fat.

13 grams of Carbs.

306 Calories.

Low-Carb Gnocchi (Serves 2)

Ingredients:

3 Egg Yolks

2 cups of Shredded Mozzarella

1/2 teaspoon of Garlic Powder

1 teaspoon of Salt

Directions:

1. Melt your mozzarella. Separate your egg yolks and beat to combine.

2. Pour 1/2 of your egg yolk mixture into your mozzarella and combine.

3. Once combined, separate it into fourths, and then roll each of these fourths into thin long strips. Do this on a piece of parchment paper.

4. Cut 1-inch pieces until you have a lot of cheese gnocchi.

5. Boil your water and drop in gnocchi. Boil them until they start to float. Remove from heat and drain out water in your strainer.

6. Fry your gnocchi on each side of your oiled pan until it is cooked.

7. Serve and Enjoy!

Nutritional Value:

28 grams of Protein.

24 grams of Fat.

4 grams of Carbs.

361 Calories.

Cabbage Fra Diavolo w/ Beef (Serves 8)

Ingredients:

24 ounces of Ground Beef (85%)

24 ounces of Pasta Sauce

1 head of Green Cabbage

1/2 cup of Water

Stick of Unsalted Butter

Pepper

Salt

Directions:

1. Remove and discard outer layer of your cabbage.

2. Quarter your cabbage and shred it in your food processor.

3. Melt your butter in large pot. Add water and cabbage. Season with pepper and salt.

4. Cook approximately 12 minutes. Stir occasionally.

5. While cooking cabbage, brown your beef.

6. Add your beef to cabbage and stir in.

7. Add pasta sauce and stir in.

8. Serve and Enjoy!

Nutritional Value - (Serving Size 8 Ounces):

19 grams of Protein.

28 grams of Fat.

11 grams of Carbs.

365 Calories.

Cauliflower Casserole (Serves 10)

Ingredients:

12 Chicken Thighs (4 ounces Each)

30 ounces of Chopped Cauliflower

8 ounces of Shredded Monterey Jack Cheese

8 ounces of Shredded Cheddar Cheese

6 Thick Cut Bacon Slices

1 medium Green Pepper

1 medium Onion

6 Green Onions

1 tablespoon of Minced Garlic

4 ounces of Heavy Cream

8 ounces of Cream Cheese

Pepper

Salt

Directions:

1. Add your chicken thighs to your casserole dish. Add pepper and salt. Add water to about mid thigh.

2. Cook for approximately 60 minutes at 350 degrees.

3 Cook you bacon at 450 degrees for 15 to 20 minutes.

4. Chop cauliflower into florets. Cook cauliflower in your microwave on the setting for vegetables.

5. Chop peppers and onions, Fry them in your pan.

6. Chop up your now cooked chicken into a big bowl.

7. Add your other ingredients except for 2 ounces of both Monterey Jack and Cheddar.

8. Add your mixture in a greased large casserole dish. Top with your remaining cheese.

9. Cover dish with foil. Cook at 350 degrees for 25 minutes. Take off foil and cook additional 5 minutes.

10. Serve and Enjoy!

Nutritional Value - (Serving Size 1/10 of Casserole):

44 grams of Protein.

34 grams of Fat.

9 grams of Carbs.

516 Calories.

Chicken Avocado Casserole (Serves 6)

Ingredients:

8 Cooked Boneless Chicken Thighs

1 medium Pepper

1 medium Onion

4 small Avocados

8 ounces of Cheddar Cheese

8 ounces of Sour Cream

1 tablespoon of Frank's Red Hot

Pepper

Salt

Directions:

1. Preheat your oven to 350 degrees.

2. If you bought chicken uncooked bake for 90 minutes at 350 degrees.

3. Peel your avocados. Cut them in half and then slice them into thinner strips.

4. Grease your baking dish. Line bottom of your dish with avocado slices.

5. Cut your onions and peppers into strips and fry in pan until it is caramelized.

6. Add your chicken to large bowl and pull apart.

7. Add in remaining ingredients.

8. Spoon your mix over your avocado slices.

9. Bake it for 20 minutes.

10. Serve and Enjoy!

Nutritional Value - (Serving Size 1/6 of Casserole):

39 grams of Protein.

40 grams of Fat.

13 grams of Carbs.

549 Calories.

Low-Carb Chicken Quesadilla (Serves 1)

Ingredients:

2.5 ounces of Grilled Chicken Breast

3 ounces of Pepper Jack

1 teaspoon of Chopped Jalapeno

1/2 Sliced Avocado

1 Low-Carb Wrap

Spices

1/4 teaspoon of Crushed Red Pepper

1/4 teaspoon of Dried Basil

1/4 teaspoon of Salt

1/4 teaspoon of Garlic Powder

Directions:

1. Grill your chopped chicken breast and spices.

2. Place your wrap on wide frying pan so it can lie flat. Cook over medium heat.

3. Cook for 2 minutes and flip your wrap over. Lay out your pepper jack. Leave less than an inch from your edges of the wrap.

4. Add your chopped chicken breast, jalapeno, and sliced avocado to 1/2 of your wrap.

5. Add your cheese.

6. Fold your wrap with your spatula and flatten by pressing down gently. You want melted cheese to glue it all together.

7. Take out of your pan and cut up into thirds. Feel free to add salsa or sour cream for dipping on the side.

8. Serve and Enjoy!

Nutritional Value:

52 grams of Protein.

43 grams of Fat.

7 grams of Carbs.

654 Calories.

Curry Chicken w/ Riced Cauliflower (Serves 6)

Ingredients:

2 pounds of Chicken (4 Breasts)

1 cup of Water

1 packet of Curry Paste

1/2 cup of Heavy Cream

3 tablespoons of Ghee

1 head of Cauliflower

Directions:

1. Melt your ghee in large pan or pot with lid.

2. Add you curry paste and stir well.

3. Once combined add your water and simmer for 5 minutes.

4. Add your chicken. Cover pan or pot and simmer for approximately 20 minutes.

5. While chicken cooks, chop your cauliflower into florets and pulse it in your food processor to make it riced cauliflower.

6. Once your chicken is cooked add in your cream and cook for 5 more minutes.

7. Place in a bowl over your riced cauliflower.

8. Serve and Enjoy!

Nutritional Value - (Serving Size 1/6 of Curry and 160 grams of Cauliflower):

38 grams of Protein.

17 grams of Fat.

10 grams of Carbs.

349 Calories.

Crispy Chicken Wings (Serves 2)

Ingredients:

12 raw Chicken Wings

4 tablespoons of Unsalted Butter

4 tablespoons of Frank's Red Hot

Directions:

1. Preheat your fryer oil to 275 degrees.

2. Pat down your wings until it is super dry.

3. Fry your wings for 14 minutes.

4. Allow wings to rest until they reach room temperature

5. Preheat your fryer to 375 degrees.

6. Pat wings dry again.

7. Fry an additional 6 minutes until they are golden brown.

8. Mix in your melted butter and Frank's Red Hot.

9. Toss your wings to coat.

10. Serve and Enjoy!

Nutritional Value - (Serving Size 6 Wings):

42 grams of Protein.

55 grams of Fat.

0 grams of Carbs.

686 Calories.

Simple Chicken Nuggets (Serves 2)

Ingredients:

1 Egg

4 ounces of Chicken Breast

2 tablespoons of Almond Flour

1/2 ounce of Grated Parmesan

1/2 teaspoon of Baking Powder

1 tablespoon of Water

Directions:

1. Heat your deep fryer to approximately 375 degrees.

2. Cook your chicken breast. Once cooked cut into cubes.

3. Mix together your almond flour, baking powder, and grated Parmesan.

4. Add your eggs and whisk.

5. Add your water and whisk.

6. Roll your chicken breast in your batter until it is fully coated. Drop them into frying oil.

7. Make sure they don't stick at the bottom of your fryer. Move them around every minute.

8. Cook for 5 minutes until your batter begins to turn golden brown.

9. Serve and Enjoy!

Nutritional Value - (Serving Size 5 Nuggets):

23 grams of Protein.

8 grams of Fat.

2 grams of Carbs.

166 Calories.

Chicken Cordon Bleu Casserole (Serves 10)

Ingredients:

53 ounces of Chicken

11 ounces of Jarlsberg Swiss Cheese

300 grams of Ham Steak

1 cup of Heavy Whipping Cream

1 cup of Cream Cheese

Garlic Powder

Pepper

Salt

Directions:

1. Cut your chicken into 1-inch cubes. Spread them out on the bottom of your pan.

2. Season with pepper, salt, and garlic powder.

3. Cut ham into 1/2 inch cubes. Sprinkle them on top of the chicken.

4. Shred your Swiss cheese and spread over top.

5. Heat your cream cheese in your microwave. Add your cream in and mix well. Pour it over casserole.

6. Bake for 40 minutes at 350 degrees.

7. Separate into 10 portions.

8. Serve and Enjoy!

Nutritional Value - (Serving Size 1/10 of Casserole):

38 grams of Protein.

30 grams of Fat.

4 grams of Carbs.

486 Calories.

Keto Lazy Chicken (Serves 2)

Ingredients:

2 Chicken Breasts

2 ounces of Jalapeno Slices

4 ounces of Cheddar Cheese

4 slices of Bacon

Pepper

Salt

Directions:

1. Season chicken with pepper and salt.

2. Cover with cheese

3. Add your jalapenos.

4. Cut your bacon in half and place over your chicken.

5. Place chicken on your foil lined pan. Bake approximately 30 to 45 minutes at 350 degrees.

6. If chicken is cooked and bacon is not quite done place under broiler for a couple minutes.

7. Serve and Enjoy!

Nutritional Value - (Serving Size 1 Chicken Breast):

70 grams of Protein.

33 grams of Fat.

1 gram of Carbs.

591 Calories.

Crockpot Buffalo Chicken (Serves 6)

Ingredients:

6 Chicken Breasts

1 bottle of Frank's Red Hot

3 tablespoons of Butter

1/2 packet of Hidden Valley Ranch

Directions:

1. Place chicken in your crockpot.

2. Pour your hot sauce over the chicken. Sprinkle your ranch over the top of it.

3. Cover it and cook over low heat for 6 hours.

4. Shred chicken, add butter and cook on low uncovered for approximately 1 hour.

5. Serve and Enjoy!

Nutritional Value - (Serving Size 1 Chicken Breast):

52 grams of Protein.

8 grams of Fat.

1 gram of Carbs.

297 Calories.

Cheesy Sausage Balls (Serves 12)

Ingredients:

6 ounces of Shredded Cheddar Cheese

12 ounces of Jimmy Dean's Sausage

12 cubes of Cheddar

Directions:

1. Mix your sausage and shredded cheese.

2. Divide up into 12 equal portions.

3. Place 1 cube of cheese into center of each sausage and roll them into balls.

4. Fry at 375 degrees until they get crispy.

5. Serve and Enjoy!

Nutritional Value - (Serving Size 1 Ball):

10 grams of Protein.

14 grams of Fat.

1 gram of Carbs.

173 Calories.

Marinated Pork Chops (Serves 10)

Ingredients:

18 Pork Chops

1/2 cup of Apple Cider Vinegar

4 tablespoons of Soy Sauce

1/2 cup of Splenda

1/2 teaspoon of Ginger

1/2 teaspoon of Pepper

Directions:

1. Add all ingredients except pork chops to your food processor.

2. Mix your marinade.

3. Put pork chops in a pan that's been greased and pour marinade on it.

4. Cook at 350 degrees for 60 minutes. Flip after approximately 30 minutes.

5. Chop your pork chops up and divide into 10 equal portions.

6. Serve and Enjoy!

Nutritional Value - (Serving Size 1/10):

46 grams of Protein.

14 grams of Fat.

1 gram of Carbs.

323 Calories.

Chapter Eight: Ketogenic Diet Dinner Recipes

In this section, I will give you 50 delicious ketogenic dinner recipes you can make yourself. I'll include both basic recipes and a few more advanced recipes. That way no matter what your level in the kitchen you'll be able to prepare healthy low carb keto meals to keep you on track with your diet. I'll add in the nutritional value whenever possible, although I don't have those exact numbers for every recipe.

Chicken Thighs w/ Spinach (Serves 8)

Ingredients:

16 Boneless Chicken Thighs (Skinless)

680 grams of Spinach

2 tablespoons of Shredded Cheddar Cheese

2 cups of Water

Garlic

Pepper

Salt

Directions:

1. Place your chicken thighs into roaster pan covered with the lid.

2. Bake at 350 degrees for 2 hours.

3. Remove and let cool.

4. Place 2 thighs each in 8 different containers.

5. Break up your thighs and place vegetables and cheese on each.

6. Distribute leftover juices over the chicken in each container.

7. Serve and Enjoy!

Nutritional Value - (Serving Size 2 Chicken Thighs):

45 grams of Protein.

23 grams of Fat.

3 grams of Carbs.

390 Calories.

Keto Chicken Divan (Serves 6)

Ingredients:

2 Boneless Chicken Breasts

1 small Yellow Onion

3 tablespoons of Ghee

1/2 teaspoon of Garlic Salt

1/2 tablespoon of Minced Garlic

Dash of Parsley

1 cup of Chicken Stock or Broth

3 cups of Cauliflower

10 cranks of Fresh Pepper

1 teaspoon of Lemon Juice

1 cup of Heavy Cream

1/2 cup of Mayonnaise

2 cups of Shredded Cheddar Cheese

3 cups of Steamed Chopped Broccoli

Directions:

1. Preheat your oven to 350 degrees.

2. Fill your pot halfway with water. Add in your chicken breasts.

3. Cook on high heat and bring to boil until your chicken is cooked.

4. Cook your onions and garlic in medium frying pan over low heat with your ghee.

5. While that cooks, blend your cauliflower using your food processor. Do this for a few seconds till it looks like rice.

6. After cooking onions for two minutes, add in your spices one by one mixing each one in.

7. Once onions are nice and soft, add in your cauliflower.

8. Once cauliflower gets soft, add in your chicken broth. Cover and cook approximately 10 minutes.

9. Take out your chicken once it's done.

10. Add in lemon juice and cream. Let it simmer uncovered over low heat for approximately 10 minutes. Mix a few times so your bottom doesn't burn.

11. Add in your mayo and mix. Turn off your burner.

12. Pull your chicken apart.

13. Add in half of your pulled chicken into cauliflower cream mix.

14. Use other 1/2 to line your 8x8 casserole dish.

15. On top of bottom chicken layer, place your steamed chopped broccoli.

16. Top with your cauliflower cream mix.

17. Top that with cheddar cheese.

18. Place in over for approximately 30 minutes. Cover it with tinfoil.

19. Remove your tinfoil and cook approximately 10 minutes.

20. Serve and Enjoy!

Loaded Baked Chicken (Serves 4)

Ingredients:

4 Chicken Breasts

1 ounce of Soy Sauce

4 Bacon Strips

4 ounces of Ranch Dressing

4 ounces of Cheddar Cheese

3 Green Onions

Directions:

1. Heat your cast iron pan and cook your oil on high heat.

2. Pan fry your chicken breasts. Flip them half way through. Total cook time should be approximately 10 to 15 minutes. Internal temperature should be 165 degrees.

3. While your chicken cooks, cook bacon and crumble into bits when done.

4. Chop up your green onions.

5. Place your chicken in your baking dish. Top it with soy sauce, then add ranch, bacon, green onions, and your cheese.

6. Broil on high for approximately 3 to 4 minutes till cheese melts.

7. Serve and Enjoy!

Nutritional Value - (Serving Size 1/4):

63 grams of Protein.

28 grams of Fat.

3 grams of Carbs.

527 Calories.

Beer Can Chicken (Serves 4)

Ingredients:

1 Whole Chicken

1 aluminum can of Beer

1 tablespoon of Bacon Fat

Rotisserie Seasoning

Directions:

1. Preheat your grill to a medium-high heat, Set it up for indirect grilling. No heat under the chicken.

2. Remove and get rid of gizzards from thawed chicken.

3. Cut away the loose skin and chicken parts from the opening of breast cavity.

4. Dry it on both outside and inside.

5. Apply oil or bacon fat to the outside of your chicken.

6. Rub in your Rotisserie seasoning on both inside and outside.

7. Remove half of beer from the can and set the chicken on the can.

8. Grill for approximately 60 minutes or until meat reads between 165 and 180 degrees.

9. Allow to rest for 5 to 10 minutes.

10. Serve and Enjoy!

Garlic Lebanese Chicken Thighs (Serves 2)

Ingredients:

4 Chicken Thighs

2 tablespoons of Ghee

Garlic Olive Oil

1 Vidalia Onion (quartered)

2 Roma Tomatoes

Handful of Baby Carrots

Oregano

15 whole cloves of Garlic

1 Juiced Fresh Lemon

Pepper

Salt

Directions:

1. Heat your oven to 500 degrees.

2. Glaze bottom of the cast iron pan with 2 teaspoons of garlic olive oil.

3. Add your 4 chicken thighs together. Make sure some space separate them.

4. Wedge your carrots, onions, tomatoes, and garlic cloves between the chicken thighs. Add two garlic cloves on the top of thighs.

5. Juice your lemon over chicken thighs.

6. Drizzle more garlic oil over top your chicken thighs.

7. Drizzle ghee over your chicken thighs.

8. Sprinkle oregano over your dish. Add pepper and salt.

9. Place in oven for approximately 30 minutes.

10. Reduce your heat to 350 degrees and then cook approximately 20 minutes till cooked to an internal temperature of 165 degrees.

11. Place your oven on broil and cook an additional 5 minutes till outside skin is crispy.

12. Remove from oven.

13. Serve and Enjoy!

Tequila Chicken (Serves 6)

Ingredients:

Marinade

6 Chicken Breasts

1 cup of Water

1/4 cup of Soy Sauce

1/2 teaspoon of Garlic Powder

2 tablespoons of Lime Juice

1/2 teaspoon of Liquid Smoke

1/2 teaspoon of Salt

1 shot of Tequila (50 ml)

Sauce

1/4 cup of Sour Cream

1/4 cup of Mayonnaise

1 tablespoon of Heavy Cream

1/4 cup of Tomato Sauce

1/4 teaspoon of Frank's Hot Sauce

1/4 teaspoon of Dried Parsley

1/4 teaspoon of Dried Dill

1/4 teaspoon of Salt

1/4 teaspoon of Paprika

1/4 teaspoon of Ground Cumin

1/4 teaspoon of Cayenne Pepper

1/4 teaspoon of Black Pepper

1/4 teaspoon of Chili Powder

6 ounces of Shredded Cheddar Cheese

Directions:

1. Mix together your marinade ingredients.

2. Add your chicken to the marinade. Let it sit and refrigerate for approximately 2 to 3 hours.

3. Place chicken on your broiler pan and then broil for approximately 20 minutes on high. Flip it after 10 minutes.

4. Check chicken for temperature. Want it to get to 165 degrees.

5. Mix ingredients for your sauce except cheese.

6. Place your meat in casserole dish. Cover it with sauce and your cheese.

7. Broil for 3 more minutes on high. Cheese should be a little bubbly.

8. Serve and Enjoy!

Nutritional Value - (Serving Size 1 Chicken Breast - Marinade not accounted for in these numbers):

60 grams of Protein.

22 grams of Fat.

2 grams of Carbs.

445 Calories.

Keto Fried Chicken (Serves 10)

Ingredients:

10 pieces of Chicken

1 cup of Crushed Pork Rinds

3/4 cup of Plain Whey Protein

1 tablespoon of Oat Fiber

1/2 teaspoon of Onion Powder

1/8 teaspoon of Coarse Black Pepper

2 large Eggs

1/2 cup of Parmesan Cheese

1/4 cup of Water

1/4 cup of Heavy Cream

3/4 inch of Deep Hot Oil

Directions:

1. Measure out and then mix together all your dry ingredients in a paper bag. Shake it well.

2. Whisk eggs, water, and cream together in a large bowl.

3. Toss in your pieces of cut up chicken into your egg mix and coat each piece completely.

4. Take pieces out of your bowl and drop in a bag of seasoned flour. When 3 pieces are in your bag, hold top closed and shake your bag to coat chicken.

5. Heat 3/4 inch deep oil on high heat.

6. Place your pieces close together. Lower the heat to medium-high. Brown chicken on one side. Turn over carefully and brown the opposite side. Should take approximately 30 minutes.

7. Remove and place on paper towel.

8. Serve and Enjoy!

Pounded Chicken Pizza (Serves 4)

Ingredients:

4 Chicken Thighs

2.5 ounces of Shredded Jarlsberg Cheese

2.5 ounces of Shredded Cheddar Cheese

1 ounce of Shredded Monterey Cheese

1/2 cup of Marinara Sauce

16 slices of Pepperoni

4 slices of Bacon

Italian Seasoning

Pepper

Salt

Directions:

1. Preheat your oven to 350 degrees.

2. Start cooking your 4 slices of bacon.

3. Place your chicken thighs on cutting board. Cover it with saran wrap. Pound it with a heavy pan.

4. Pepper and salt both sides of your chicken.

5. Heat up grease in your pan over high heat. Sear your chicken on each side for one minute.

6. Transfer skillet to your oven and cook approximately 10 minutes.

7. Remove skillet from oven. Add your seasoning and sauce.

8. Cover it with cheese and place back in your oven for approximately 3 minutes on broil.

9. Remove from oven. Add your remaining toppings. This includes pepperoni and bacon. Broil for 2 more minutes.

10. Serve and Enjoy!

Nutritional Value - (Serving Size 1 Chicken Thigh):

32 grams of Protein.

36 grams of Fat.

1 gram of Carbs.

461 Calories.

Beer Can Burgers (Serves 5)

Ingredients:

50 ounces of Ground Beef

2.5 ounces of Pepper Jack Cheese (cubed)

2.5 ounces of Shredded Extra Sharp Cheddar Cheese

10 slices of Bacon

150 grams of cooked Brussels Sprouts

150 grams of cooked Sliced Fresh Mushrooms

150 grams of cooked Onions

150 grams of cooked Green Peppers

Directions:

1. Preheat your grill to 300 degrees. Set it up for indirect heat.

2. Divide your ground beef into equal amounts and make them into large balls.

3. Push a can into your ball and smush it.

4. Using your own hand, for meat around the can, making sure to push it up evenly around your can.

5. Wrap 2 pieces of bacon around the base of your meat.

6. Extract your can and fill the hole with whatever you'd like. In this example, we used green peppers, onions, Brussels sprouts, and mushrooms.

7. Top it with some cheese.

8. Place on your grill and cook with indirect heat for approximately 1 hour.

9. Take off your grill.

10. Serve and Enjoy!

Nutritional Value - (Serving Size 1 Burger):

66 grams of Protein.

73 grams of Fat.

8 grams of Carbs.

963 Calories.

Juicy Sliders (Serves 4)

Ingredients:

1 Egg

1 pound of Ground Beef

8 ounces of Cheddar Cheese

Dash of Worcestershire Sauce

Garlic

Onion Powder

Pepper

Salt

Directions:

1. Mix your eggs, spices, and beef.

2. Divide your meat into patties of 1.5 ounces.

3. Add a 1/2 ounce of cheese to each of your patties.

4. Combine two of your patties to form one burger. Use your hands to meld the two patties together.

5. Heat oil on high and then fry your burgers to your desired level.

6. Top with cheese and your desired toppings.

Nutritional Value - (Serving Size 1 Slider):

22 grams of Protein.

21 grams of Fat.

0 grams of Carbs.

285 Calories.

Bacon Wrapped Brats (Serves 4)

Ingredients:

4 Bacon Slices

4 Brats

4 slices of Cheese

2 12 ounce Beers

4 Romaine Lettuce Leafs

Directions:

1. Place your brats in your pot. Cover it with your beer.

2. Boil approximately 10 minutes.

3. Remove your brats and wrap with your bacon.

4. Grill your bacon wrapped brats till bacon gets crisp.

5. Serve and Enjoy!

Flank Steak Pinwheels (Serves 6)

Ingredients:

2 pounds of Flank Steak

8 ounces of Fresh Spinach

16 ounces of Mozzarella Cheese

Italian Seasoning

Directions:

1. Preheat your oven to 350 degrees.

2. Place flank steak so your grain is going right to left.

3. Square your flank and remove hard fat deposits.

4. Using a sharp knife, butterfly your steak. Be sure to cut parallel to your cutting board leaving about an inch not cut. Always cut along the grain.

5. Open your steak, using your knife to finish off the cut so a 1/2 is still connected.

6. Lay steak flat. Grain needs to be facing up and down your cutting board.

7. Season each side with Italian seasoning.

8. Spread your mozzarella cheese over steak. Leave an inch on one of your sides for wrapping.

9. Lay down two layers of spinach.

10. Roll your steak. Be sure to keep it tight, rolling it with your grain.

11. Cut 6 pieces of twine and then tie off 6 sections spaced evenly.

12. Cut out your pinwheels carefully by cutting between twine pieces.

13. Place in your Pyrex baking dish over a layer of spinach.

14. Cook approximately 25 minutes.

15. Broil for about 3 minutes till cheese is bubbly.

16. Serve and Enjoy!

Nutritional Value - (Serving Size 1/6):

57 grams of Protein.

29 grams of Fat.

1 gram of Carbs.

519 Calories.

Fat Burning Ginger Steak (Serves 2)

Ingredients:

2 Sirloin Steaks (each 4 ounces)

1 Diced Small Onion

1 crushed clove of Garlic

1 tablespoon of Olive Oil

2 small Diced Tomatoes

4 tablespoons Apple Cider Vinegar

1 teaspoon of Ground Ginger

Pepper

Salt

Directions:

1. Place your oil in large skillet. Brown your steaks over a medium-high heat.

2. Once each side seared, add in your tomatoes, garlic, and onion.

3. In your bowl, add salt, pepper, ginger into vinegar and then add your mixture to your skillet. Stir well to combine.

4. Cover your skillet, turn heat to low and allow to simmer to your liquids are completely evaporated.

5. Serve and Enjoy!

Nutritional Value - (Serving Size 1 Steak):

31 grams of Protein.

8 grams of Fat.

3 grams of Carbs.

208 Calories.

Stuffed & Seared Flank Steak (Serves 6)

Ingredients:

2 Flank Steaks

7 ounces of Roasted Red Peppers

16 ounces of Spinach

4 ounces of Bleu Cheese

1 Egg Yolk

2 tablespoons of Almond Flour

1/2 teaspoon of Onion Powder

1/2 teaspoon of Garlic Powder

1/2 teaspoon of Salt

1/2 teaspoon of Pepper

Directions:

1. Place grain of your flank steak vertically.

2. Butterfly steak cutting from right to left.

3. Microwave your frozen spinach and then drain any liquid.

4. Slice your roasted red peppers.

5. Combine your remaining ingredients with your spinach. Mix well.

6. Spread your mixture over your steak and then roll with your grain.

7. Truss your steak with some cotton twine.

8. Wrap it with saran wrap. Marinate it for approximately 30 minutes.

9. Cook for approximately 35 minutes at 425 degrees.

10. Broil steak for 10 minutes. Rotate steak after approximately 5 minutes.

11. Cover it with your foil. Rest for 10 minutes.

12. Serve and Enjoy!

Nutritional Value - (Serving Size 1/6):

54 grams of Protein.

25 grams of Fat.

6 grams of Carbs.

470 Calories.

Bacon Wrapped Filet Mignon w/ Bleu Cheese Butter (Serves 8)

Ingredients:

<u>Bacon Wrapped Filet Mignon</u>

8 Filet Mignon Steaks. (8 to 10 ounces each. 3-inch thick cut)

8 slices of Bacon

Pepper

Salt

<u>Bleu Cheese Butter</u>

2 tablespoons of Minced Garlic

Stick of Butter

1/4 teaspoon of Montreal Steak Seasoning

1/4 teaspoon of Onion Powder

1/4 teaspoon of Dried Thyme

Directions:

<u>Bleu Cheese Butter</u>

1. Soften your butter. Once soft add to your food processor.

2. Add rest of the bleu cheese butter ingredients except bleu cheese.

3. Mince your mixture until it is blended.

4. Add your bleu cheese and mix well.

5. Transfer to container and refrigerate.

Bacon Wrapped Filet Mignon

1. Bring meat to room temperature. Should take approximately 30 minutes.

2. Pepper and salt both sides.

3. Wrap your bacon and secure it with a toothpick.

4. Sear it on high heat. Do so in an oven proof skillet. Sear for 3 minutes on both sides.

5. Transfer to your oven and set at 450 degrees.

6. Should take approximately 8 to 10 minutes to cook for each steak. Check meat for desired preference. I like mine medium well.

Nutritional Value - (Serving Size 9 Ounces):

61 grams of Protein.

37 grams of Fat.

1 grams of Carbs.

598 Calories.

Steak w/ Mushroom Port Sauce (Serves 2)

Ingredients:

2 pounds of Rib Eye Steak

2 ounces of Heavy Cream

10 ounces of Mushrooms

1 tablespoon of Butter

4 ounces of Port Wine

Pepper

Salt

Directions:

1. Preheat your oven to 450 degrees.

2. Pepper and salt each side of steak.

3. Heat your cast iron skillet on high heat.

4. Melt your butter until it bubbles.

5. Cook steak approximately 2 minutes on each side and then move to your oven for finishing.

6. Cook in your oven until the internal temperature is above 135 degrees. The higher the temp the more well done it will be. Should take about 12 minutes. Be sure to flip steaks at the 6-minute mark.

7. Once steaks are finished remove from oven and cover with some foil.

8. Add your port wine to a pan to deglaze. Scrap the bits of burnt stuff from the bottom.

9. Add your cream and mushrooms. Light on fire.

10. Once your sauce has got thicker, pour it over steak.

11. Serve and Enjoy!

Nutritional Value - (Serving Size 1 Steak):

102 grams of Protein.

62 grams of Fat.

6 grams of Carbs.

984 Calories.

Parmesan Encrusted Pork Chops (Serves 14)

Ingredients:

14 Bone-In Pork Chops

2 large Eggs

3/4 cup of Almond Flour

6 ounces of Parmesan Cheese

Pepper

Salt

Directions:

1. Grate your Parmesan cheese and combine it with almond flour and spices.

2. Whisk your eggs and put in a shallow container.

3. Dip your pork chops in your eggs and coat with Parmesan mix.

4. Fry pork chops in bacon grease in your pan for 1 minute on each side.

5. Cook at 400 degrees in your oven for approximately 10 minutes or until it is done to desired preference. The amount of time will depend on the thickness of your pork chops.

6. Serve and Enjoy!

Nutritional Value - (Serving Size 1 Pork Chop):

33 grams of Protein.

34 grams of Fat.

4 grams of Carbs.

454 Calories.

Pan Fried Pork Chops (Serves 3)

Ingredients:

3 Bone-In Pork Chops

1 teaspoon of Black Pepper

1 teaspoon of Seasoned Salt

1/2 cup of Coconut Flour

1 tablespoon of Butter

1/4 teaspoon of Cayenne Pepper

Directions:

1. Mix all your dry ingredients together in a container big enough to fit your pork chops.

2. Dry pork chops.

3. Heat your skillet on high. Add in butter.

4. Coat your pork chops in the dry mix and fry.

5. Cook approximately 5 minutes per side until it is done to your preference.

6. Serve and Enjoy!

Nutritional Value - (Serving Size 1 Pork Chop):

27 grams of Protein.

15 grams of Fat.

11 grams of Carbs.

298 Calories.

Keto Asian Pork Chops (Serves 2)

Ingredients:

4 Boneless Pork Chops

1 stalk of Lemon Grass (diced and peeled)

1 medium Star Anise

1 tablespoon of Almond Flour

1 tablespoon of Fish Sauce

4 halved Garlic Cloves

1/2 tablespoon of Sambal Chili Paste

1/2 tablespoon of Sugar-Free Ketchup

1 1/2 teaspoons of Soy Sauce

1/2 teaspoon of Five Spice

1 teaspoon of Sesame Oil

1/2 teaspoon of Peppercorns

Directions:

1. Place chops on a flat surface and use your rolling pin wrapped in some wax paper to pound chops to 1/2 inch thickness.

2. Cut garlic cloves in half.

3. Grind your star anise and peppercorns to a fine powder using your blender. Add in garlic and lemon grass. Blend until in puree form. Add your soy sauce, fish sauce, five-spice, and sesame oil. Mix it together well.

4. Place pork chops on a tray and pour on your marinade. Coat on both sides. Cover and let marinate at room temperature approximately 2 hours.

5. Sear pork chops on both sides in your pan. Should take approximately 2 minutes on both sides. Should see a golden brown crust forming.

6. Transfer over to your cutting board and cut each of the chops into strips.

7. To make your sauce, stir your Sambal chili paste and ketchup together.

8. Serve and Enjoy!

Nutritional Values - (Serving Size 1/2):

34 grams of Protein.

9.5 grams of Fat.

6 grams of Carbs.

272 Calories.

Blackened Pork Chops (Serves 4)

Ingredients:

4 Pork Chops

2 teaspoon of Salt

1 tablespoon of Paprika

2 teaspoon of Salt

1 teaspoon of Onion Powder

1 teaspoon of Garlic Powder

2 teaspoon of Black Pepper

1/4 teaspoon of Cayenne Pepper

1/2 teaspoon of Oregano Leaves

1/2 teaspoon of Thyme Leaves

4 tablespoons of Butter

1 teaspoon of Cumin

Directions:

1. Assemble your spices and mix it in a shallow bowl big enough to fit pork chop.

2. Melt your butter in a different bowl.

3. Heat up some bacon grease in your skillet.

4. Dip your chops in butter and coat with your spices. Put it in the oil.

5. Cook approximately 3 to 5 minutes per side.

6. Flip once and cook until the temperature reaches between 140 to 150 degrees.

7. Serve and Enjoy!

Nutritional Value - (Serving Size 1 Pork Chop):

46 grams of Protein.

15 grams of Fat.

4 grams of Carbs.

341 Calories.

Stuffed Pork Chops (Serves 4)

Ingredients:

4 Thick Cut Pork Chops

3 ounces of Feta Cheese

3 ounces of Bleu Cheese

3 slices of Bacon

2 ounces of Cream Cheese

60 grams of Green Onion

Garlic

Pepper

Salt

Directions:

1. Cook your bacon in a skillet. Reserve grease and put bacon aside.

2.. Combine your feta and bleu cheese in a bowl.

3. Add green onions and bacon. Mix well.

4. Add your cream cheese and mix it until well combined.

5. Slice open nonfatty side of pork chop.

6. Stuff it with your cheese mixture.

7. Use toothpick to close the opening.

8. Apply your pepper, garlic powder, and salt to the outside of the pork chops.

9. Over some high heat with your bacon grease in the pan, sear each chop for 1.5 minutes per side.

10. Transfer your chops to greased pan. Cook for approximately 55 minutes at 350 degrees.

11. Remove chops and allow to rest for 3 minutes.

12. Serve and Enjoy!

Nutritional Value - (Serving Size 1 Pork Chop):

102 grams of Protein.

38 grams of Fat.

2 grams of Carbs.

778 Calories.

Italian Parmesan Pork Cutlets (Serves 6)

Ingredients:

6 Pork Cutlets

1/2 cup of Grated Parmesan Cheese

1/2 cup of Italian Dressing

Seasonings of your choice.

Directions:

1. Heat your frying pan over medium heat.

2. Pour Italian dressing in your bowl.

3. Pour your grated Parmesan cheese in a bowl.

4. Dip cutlets first in Italian dressing and then in your Parmesan cheese.

5. Cook cutlets for approximately 15 minutes in your pan.

6. Serve and Enjoy!

Bacon & Beef Rolls (Serves 4)

Ingredients:

16 ounces of Beef

4 slices of Bacon

Montreal Steak Seasoning

Directions:

1. Preheat your oil in a deep fryer to approximately 370 degrees.

2. Cut your beef into 1 x 1 x 2-inch cubes. Should weigh 1 ounce each.

3. Take bacon and stretch it. Cut each piece into 4 smaller pieces.

4. Season your meat with the Montreal steak seasoning.

5. Wrap your beef with some bacon and skewer.

6. Cook approximately 3 minutes in your deep fryer.

7. Serve and Enjoy!

Nutritional Value - (Serving Size 4 Pieces):

29 grams of Protein.

10 grams of Fat.

0 grams of Carbs.

215 Calories.

Bacon Wrapped Sausages (Serves 4)

Ingredients:

10 slices of Bacon

5 Italian Chicken Sausages

Directions:

1. Preheat your deep fryer to 370 degrees.

2. Cut each of your sausages into four pieces.

3. Cut the bacon in half.

4. Wrap your bacon over your sausage covering up the cut end.

5. Skewer your bacon and sausage.

6. Fry it for approximately 3 to 4 minutes.

7. Serve and Enjoy!

Nutritional Value - (Serving Size 5 Pieces):

25 grams of Protein.

18 grams of Fat.

2 grams of Carbs.

273 Calories.

Keto St. Louis Ribs

Ingredients:

2 racks of St. Louis Ribs

2 tablespoons of Splenda

2 tablespoons of Paprika

1 tablespoon of Garlic Powder

1/2 tablespoon of Pepper

1 tablespoon of Salt

2 ounces of Dijon Mustard

1/2 tablespoon of Onion Powder

1/2 tablespoon of Ground Ginger

1/4 tablespoon of Cayenne Pepper

Directions:

1. Preheat your oven to 225 degrees.

2. Remove membrane from back of your ribs.

3. Mix your spices together.

4. Spread mustard over all your ribs.

5. Rub your spice mix into meat.

6. Place your ribs on foil-lined baking sheet.

7. Bake it uncovered for approximately 60 minutes.

8. Tent your meat with some aluminum foil. Cook approximately 3.5 hours. Turn after about 2 hours.

9. Remove your foil and then broil it approximately 5 minutes to help develop a nice crust.

10. Cover it and allow to rest for 10 minutes.

11. Serve and Enjoy!

Nutritional Value - (Serving Size 4 Ribs):

99 grams of Protein.

59 grams of Fat.

4 grams of Carbs.

925 Calories.

Zoodles w/ Lamb Meatballs (Serves 4)

Ingredients:

1 pound of Ground Lamb

16 ounces of Pasta Sauce

1 pound of Zoodles (used 2 pound Zucchini)

1 Yolk

2 Shallots

1 teaspoon of Cumin

1 teaspoon of Cinnamon

Cayenne Pepper

Red Pepper Flakes

Pepper

Salt

Directions:

1. Preheat your oven to 450 degrees.

2. Use a mandoline with julienne setting and slice your zucchini into zoodles. Only slice outer parts. Stop when you reach the seeds.

3. Mix rest of your ingredients besides pasta sauce. Form 16 1 ounce meatballs.

4. Cook your meatballs approximately 12 minutes.

5. Add your sauce and zoodles to a saucepan and cook approximately 3 to 4 minutes.

6. Serve and Enjoy!

Nutritional Value - (Serving Size 1/4):

23 grams of Protein.

30 grams of Fat.

13 grams of Carbs.

426 Calories.

Crockpot Chorizo & Chicken Soup (Serves 8)

Ingredients:

4 pounds of Boneless Skinless Chicken Thighs

4 cups of Chicken Stock

1 pound of Chorizo

1 can of Stewed Tomatoes

1 cup of Heavy Cream

2 tablespoons of Worcestershire Sauce

2 tablespoons of Minced Garlic

2 tablespoons of Frank's Hot Sauce

Shaved Parmesan

Sour Cream

Directions:

1. Brown your chorizo in a skillet.

2. Layer your ingredients in your crockpot starting with raw chicken thighs, then chorizo and then the remaining ingredients except sour cream and shaved parmesan.

3. Cook for approximately 3 hours on high.

4. Remove your thighs, break them apart, and place back in your crockpot.

5. Cook approximately 30 minutes on low heat.

6. Garnish with sour cream and shaved parmesan.

Nutritional Value - (Serving Size 1/8):

52 grams of Protein.

47 grams of Fat.

6 grams of Carbs.

659 Calories.

Roasted Duck (Serves 4)

Ingredients:

1 Duck

Directions:

1. Thaw your duck. Remove any excess fat. Remove extras like the neck, heart, and liver.

2. Tie the duck legs together.

3. Cook for 3 hours at approximately 300 degrees. Turn and poke with your knife every 30 minutes. Poke through the skin but don't penetrate the meat. After 25 pokes you should see the fat oozing out of where you poked.

4. Once finished take out of the oven and quarter your roasted duck.

5. Serve and Enjoy!

Nutritional Value - (Serving Size 1/4):

38 grams of Protein.

38 grams of Fat.

0 grams of Carbs.

495 Calories.

Sous Vide Prime Rib

Ingredients:

5 Pounds of Prime Rib

Pepper

Salt

Directions:

1. Salt and pepper your meat.

2. Set your sous vide to 58 C.

3. Vacuum seal your prime rib.

4. Cook approximately 10 hours.

5. Broil your finished prime rib for a few minutes.

6. Serve and Enjoy!

Sunflower Butter Pork Kabobs (Serves 4)

Ingredients:

1 pound of Pork Kabob Square

3 tablespoons of Sunflower Butter

2 teaspoons of Hot Sauce

1 tablespoon of Minced Garlic

1 tablespoon of Soy Sauce

1/2 teaspoon of Crushed Red Pepper

1 medium Green Pepper

1 tablespoon of Water

Directions:

1. Place your marinade ingredients in your small food processor and mix till smooth.

2. Cut your pork up into bite size squares. Place these in your non-metal bowl.

3. Mix your marinade and pork together. Allow to marinate at least 1 hour but not for more than a day.

4. Chop up green pepper into smaller pieces.

5. Thread your pork and green pepper onto your metal skewers.

6. Broil on each side for approximately 5 minutes on high. Internal temperature should reach at least 145 degrees.

7. Serve and Enjoy!

<u>Nutritional Value - (Serving Size 1 Kabob):</u>

24 grams of Protein.

8 grams of Fat.

5 grams of Carbs.

200 Calories.

Creamy Chicken w/ Spaghetti Squash (Serves 4)

Ingredients:

12 ounces of chicken

5 ounces of Spinach

14 ounces of Spaghetti Squash

4 ounces of Cream Cheese

1 tablespoon of Minced Garlic

1 ounce of Grated Parmesan Cheese

Directions:

1. Make your spaghetti squash. A have a recipe for it earlier in the book.

2. Dice and then cook your 12 ounces of chicken.

3. Microwave your spinach until it is thawed and drain any excess liquid.

4. Heat up bacon grease in your cast iron skillet

5. Add your spaghetti squash and your spinach. Saute it.

6. Add in your chicken.

7. Add your Parmesan cheese and cream cheese. Mix well.

8. Top with additional Parmesan cheese once cooked.

9. Serve and Enjoy!

Nutritional Value - (Serving Size 1/4):

33 grams of Protein.

15 grams of Fat.

9 grams of Carbs.

308 Calories.

BBQ Pot Roast (Serves 12)

Ingredients:

8 pounds of Beef Chuck Shoulder Roast

5 teaspoons of Minced Garlic

1 Yellow Onion

3 tablespoons of Bacon Grease or Butter

4 tablespoons of Vinegar

2 tablespoons of Worcestershire Sauce

4 tablespoons of Splenda

1 tablespoon of Yellow Mustard

1 teaspoon of Liquid Smoke

Pepper

Salt

Directions:

1. Rough chop your onion and set to the side.

2. Coat your roast with pepper and salt.

3. Heat up your bacon grease in a pan and sear roast on each side. Approximately 1.5 minutes each side.

4. Place meat in your crockpot.

5. Fry your onions in leftover grease. Pour this over your meat.

6. Mix together your garlic, mustard, Splenda, vinegar, liquid smoke, and Worcestershire sauce.

7. Pour this sauce over your meat.

8. Cook on low in your crockpot approximately 1 hour and 15 minutes per each pound of roast. I cooked this one approximately 9 hours.

9. Remove your roast from your crockpot. Separate into 12 equal portions.

10.. Move your liquid to your pan and reduce it by half. Serve this with your meat.

11. Serve and Enjoy!

Nutritional Value - (Serving Size 1/12):

75 grams of Protein.

22 grams of Fat.

4 grams of Carbs.

701 Calories.

Bacon Wrapped Scallops (Serves 3)

Ingredients:

12 Thin Bacon Slices

12 Scallops

1 tablespoon of Oil

Pepper

Salt

12 Toothpicks

Directions:

1. Heat skillet on high heat with oil.

2. Wrap each of your scallops with bacon and secure with your toothpick.

3. Season with pepper and salt.

4. Cook 2 1/2 minutes on each side.

5. Serve and Enjoy!

Nutritional Value - (Serving Size 4 Scallops):

27 grams of Protein.

10 grams of Fat.

3 grams of Carbs.

204 Calories.

Bacon Explosion (Serves 10)

Ingredients:

14 ounces of Steak

29 slices of Thick Cut Bacon

4 ounces of Shredded Cheddar Cheese

10 ounces of Pork Sausage

Directions:

1. Layout a 5 x 6 bacon weave in baking dish. Bake for approximately 15 to 20 minutes at 400 degrees until nearly crisp.

2. Create your meat mixture by grinding the bacon, sausage, and steak.

3. Layout your meat in a rectangle that was the size of the first bacon weave.

4. Season your meat and then place your bacon weave on your meat.

5. Place your cheese in the center of the bacon.

6. Roll your meat into a right roll. Place in refrigerator for a little bit.

7. Make a 7 x7 bacon wave over your meat in a diagonal pattern.

8. Bake for 50 to 60 minutes at 400 degrees. Internal temperature should reach 165 degrees.

9. Allow to rest for 10 minutes.

10. Serve and Enjoy!

Nutritional Value - (Serving Size 1/10):

29 grams of Protein.

26 grams of Fat.

1 gram of Carbs.

353 Calories.

Stuffed Peppers (Serves 2)

Ingredients:

1 Egg

2 Green Peppers

2 Quail Eggs

1 Small Onion

1.5 ounces of Parmesan Cheese

2 Sausage Links

2 ounces of Cream Cheese

Directions:

1. Remove skin from sausage and then cook your sausage into crumbles.

2. Cut off top of your peppers and remove their seeds.

3. Chop your onions. Cook both onions and peppers.

4. Chop the Parmesan cheese into little pieces.

5. Combine onions, peppers, cheese, cream cheese, and sausage.

6. Stuff your peppers with your stuffing and then top it with a quail egg.

7. Cook at 400 degrees for approximately 20 minutes.

8. Serve and Enjoy!

Nutritional Value - (Serving Size 1 Pepper):

30 grams of Protein.

35 grams of Fat.

14 grams of Carbs.

484 Calories.

Meat Pizza (Serves 4)

Ingredients:

2 large Eggs

20 ounces of Ground Beef

28 Pepperoni Slices

1/2 cup of Shredded Cheddar Cheese

1/2 cup of Pizza Sauce

4 ounces of Mozzarella Cheese

Garlic Powder

Pepper

Salt

Directions:

1. Mix your ground beef, seasoning, and eggs together.

2. Put your ground beef into a cast iron skillet. Form it into a pizza crust.

3. Cook at 400 degrees for approximately 15 minutes.

4. Take out your crust and add your sauce, cheese, then toppings.

5. Cook until your cheese is completely melted.

6. Serve and Enjoy!

Nutritional Value - (Serving Size 1/4):

44 grams of Protein.

45 grams of Fat.

3 grams of Carbs.

610 Calories.

Sausage & Banana Pepper Fried Pizza (Serves 1)

Ingredients:

1 1/2 cups of Mozzarella Cheese

1 tablespoon of Garlic Infused Olive Oil

1/3 cup of Tomato Sauce

Italian Seasoning

Grated Parmesan Cheese

<u>Toppings</u>

1/4 cup of Mozzarella Cheese

Chopped Yellow Onions

Cooked Crumbled Sausage

Chopped Banana Peppers

Directions:

1. Preheat your broiler to 500 degrees.

2. Heat a non-stick pan over medium heat and add in your garlic oil.

3. When the oil has coated your pan, add in the mozzarella cheese.

4. Use your spatula to evenly spread the cheese and round any corners like you would a pizza.

5. Cook approximately 3 to 5 minutes while cheese melts and begins to get dark around edges.

6. Once your cheese is melted add your tomato sauce gently with a spoon.

7. Cook for about 1 more minute.

8. Use your spatula and slide around edges of your pizza and underneath to de-stick it from your pan. Don't lift it off.

9. Once your pizza is free from your pan, tip pan and slide pizza onto a pan lined with foil. Use a spatula to guide it.

10. Sprinkle with Italian seasonings and grated cheese.

11. Top with 1/4 cup of mozzarella cheese, banana peppers, sausage, and onions.

12. Place in oven approximately 2 minutes till toppings get hot.

13. Allow to sit for 2 minutes while your cheese hardens and begins to become like a crust.

14. Serve and Enjoy!

Roasted Leg of Lamb (Serves 6)

Ingredients:

3 pounds of Boneless Leg of Lamb

2 tablespoons of Minced Garlic

Twine

1 teaspoon of Rosemary

1 teaspoon of Thyme

1 tablespoon of Lemon Juice

1/2 teaspoon of Pepper

1 tablespoon of Olive Oil

2 tablespoons of Butter

1/2 cup of Dry Red Wine

Directions:

1. Preheat your oven to 450 degrees.

2. Trim fat off the fatty side of your lamb leg.

3. Add crisscross pattern onto fat side of your roast.

4. Mix spices in small bowl. Apply mix to each side of roast.

5. Using twine, truss your leg of lamb so it's closed.

6. Place it on your roasting pan and cook for approximately 15 minutes at 450 degrees.

7. After about 15 minutes, turn heat down to 325 degrees and then cook for 45 more minutes.

8. Let your meat rest about 5 minutes.

9. Add wine to your pan and then deglaze it.

10. Remove the twine and slice.

11. Serve and Enjoy!

Nutritional Value - (Serving Size 1/6):

40 grams of Protein.

44 grams of Fat.

3 grams of Carbs.

594 Calories.

Bourbon Glazed Ham (Serves 12)

Ingredients:

Ham:

8 to 12 Pound Bone-in Ham Shank

Glaze:

2 ounces of Bourbon

1 1/4 cup of Splenda

1 teaspoon of Champagne Vinegar

1 teaspoon of Ground Mustard

Cloves

Directions:

1. Trim the fat and then crisscross your ham.

2. Place it in your roasting pan. Add water an inch or two high and cover. Cook approximately 1 hour at 325 degrees.

3. Prepare your glaze combining all ingredients except your cloves.

4. After an hour, drain most of your water from roasting pan.

5. Apply your glaze and place your cloves in the crisscross areas.

6. Cook approximately 1 hour uncovered.

7. Serve and Enjoy!

Nutritional Value - (Serving Size 1/12):

50 grams of Protein.

32 grams of Fat.

6 grams of Carbs.

548 Calories.

Mac N Cheese Spaghetti Squash (Serves 6)

Ingredients:

3 Spaghetti Squash

12 ounces of Aged Cheddar

1/4 cup of Heavy Cream

2 ounces of Parmesan

4 ounces of Cheddar

1 Small Onion

1 Medium Pepper

Directions:

1. Prepare your spaghetti squash per the recipe earlier in this book.

2. Slice your onions and pepper thinly.

3. Heat your cream in a big pot and add in your cheese.

4. Stir your cheese till it combines with cream and gets smooth.

5. Add your vegetables and noodles. Mix together well.

6. Transfer mixture to greased casserole dish. Bake at 350 degrees approximately 25 minutes.

7. Serve and Enjoy!

Nutritional Values - (Serving Size 1/6):

22 grams of Protein.

29 grams of Fat.

16 grams of Carbs.

405 Calories.

Reuben Casserole (Serves 4)

Ingredients:

12 ounces of Cooked Corned Beef

1 Small Onion

8 ounces of Jarlsberg

1 can of Sauerkraut

4 ounces of Cheddar Cheese

1/4 cup of Mayo

1/2 cup of Thousand Island Dressing

Pepper

Directions:

1. Slice and dice corned beef. Add it to a big bowl.

2. Use a grater with a big opening, shred your onion, add it to your bowl.

3. Use the same grater on Jarlsberg, add it to your bowl.

4. Drain your can of Sauerkraut, add it to your bowl.

5. Add your cheddar cheese to your bowl.

6. Add your mayo and Thousand Island dressing to the bowl.

7. Add some fresh pepper.

8. Mix together and spread into your 8-inch greased pan.

9. Cook for 35 minutes at 350 degrees.

10. Serve and Enjoy!

<u>Nutritional Value - (Serving Size 1/4):</u>

37 grams of Protein.

63 grams of Fat.

10 grams of Carbs.

769 Calories.

Crockpot Corned Beef & Cabbage (Serves 10)

Ingredients:

6 pounds of Corned Beef

4 cups of Water

1 Celery Bunch

1 Small Onion

4 Carrots

1/2 teaspoon of Ground Mustard

1/2 teaspoon of Ground Coriander

1/2 teaspoon of Salt

1/2 teaspoon of Black Pepper

1/2 teaspoon of Allspice

1/2 teaspoon of Ground Thyme

1 Large Cabbage Head

1/2 teaspoon of Ground Marjoram

Directions:

1. Cut up your celery, carrots, and onions.

2. Line your crockpot with vegetables.

3. Add your water.

4. Mix your spices all together.

5. Rub each side of corned beef with your spices and put on top of vegetables.

6. Cover and then cook in crockpot on low for 7 hours.

7. Discard top layer of your cabbage. Wash and then quarter.

8. Put cabbage in crockpot. Cook for another hour on low.

9. Serve and Enjoy!

Nutritional Value - (Serving Size 1/10):

42 grams of Protein.

40 grams of Fat.

13 grams of Carbs.

583 Calories.

Kimchi Shirataki Noodles (Serves 4)

Ingredients:

2 House Foods Tofu Shirataki Noodles

1/2 container of Kimchi

4 ounces of Sliced Pork Belly

1 tablespoon of Sesame Oil

1 tablespoon of Fish Sauce

1 tablespoon of Soy Sauce

4 stalks of Green Onions

Directions:

1. Prep your ingredients.

2. Cut pork belly into small bit size pieces.

3. Cut kimchi into smaller bite size pieces.

4. Wash your noodles.

5. Add your oils to wok and heat it on high.

6. Add your pork belly and fry it for a few minutes until it's cooked.

7. Throw in your kimchi and continue to fry it.

8. Make a hole in the middle of your wok. Add your noodles. Fry till hot.

9. Transfer to bowl and top it with your green onions.

10. Serve and Enjoy!

Nutritional Value - (Serving Size 1/4):

6 grams of Protein.

19 grams of Fat.

6 grams of Carbs.

221 Calories.

Mahi-Mahi w/ Hummus (Serves 1)

Ingredients:

1 Mahi Mahi Filet

1 cup of Frozen Vegetables

2 tablespoons of Hummus

1 tablespoon of Lime

1 teaspoon of Philadelphia Cheese

Fresh Coriander

Ground Pepper

Sea Salt

Cilantro

Directions :

1. Place your vegetables on the bottom basket and your Mahi Mahi on top basket.

2. Add your lime, pepper, salt, and cilantro.

3. Set your steamer for approximately 30 minutes.

4. Add cheese on your vegetables and hummus as a side dish.

5. Serve and Enjoy!

Nutritional Value:

35 grams of Protein.

7 grams of Fat.

10 grams of Carbs.

228 Calories.

Coconut Shrimp & Avocado (Serves 1)

Ingredients:

1 cup of Shrimp

1/2 tablespoon of Organic Peanut Butter

1/2 half of an Avocado

1 tablespoon of Light Coconut Milk

1 teaspoon of Shredded Coconut

Sriracha Hot Sauce

Olive Oil

Directions:

1. Set a non-stick saute pan over medium heat. Spray with olive oil.

2. Pour in the Sriracha, coconut milk, and peanut butter.

3. Add your shrimp and saute approximately 3 to 4 minutes till shrimps turn pink.

4. Cut your half of an avocado into cubes and place on a plate.

5. Add your shrimps on the top of the avocado and sprinkle with your shredded coconut.

6. Serve and Enjoy!

Nutritional Value:

24 grams of Protein.

12 grams of Fat.

11 grams of Carbs.

250 Calories.

Keto Baked Salmon

Ingredients:

2 pounds of Salmon Fillets

1/2 cup of Tamari Soy Sauce

4 ounces of Sesame Oil

1 teaspoon of Minced Garlic

1/2 teaspoon of Basil

1/2 teaspoon of Ground Ginger

1/2 teaspoon of Rosemary

1/4 teaspoon of Thyme

1/2 teaspoon of Rosemary

1 teaspoon of Oregano Leaves

1/4 teaspoon of Tarragon

4 ounces of Butter

1/2 cup of Chopped Green Onions

1/2 cup of Chopped Fresh Mushrooms

Directions:

1. Cut fillet into 1/2 pound pieces. Get out a 1-quart freezer Ziploc bag.

2. Stir together your spices, sesame oil, and tamari sauce. Put your salmon in a Ziploc bag and then pour in your sauce mix.

3. Refrigerate your salmon with the skin side facing up in your marinade for 1 to 4 hours.

4. Preheat your oven to 350 degrees. Line with foil a large sized baking pan.

5. Pour out your fillets and marinade into your pan. Lay out your fish in a single layer.

6. Bake your fillets for approximately 10 to 15 minutes.

7. While salmon cooks prepare your vegetables.

8. Melt your butter. Add your vegetables to it and mix to coat your vegetables.

9. Remove salmon from oven and pour your butter mixture over salmon so each one is covered.

10. Bake for 10 more minutes at 350 degrees.

11. Serve and Enjoy!

Nutritional Value - (Serving Size 8 oz):

32 grams of Protein.

23 grams of Fat.

2 grams of Carbs.

353 Calories.

Keto Meatloaf (Serves 12)

Ingredients:

1 pound of Italian Sausage

2 pounds of 85% Ground Beef

2 Large Eggs

8 ounces of Chopped White Onion

1/2 cup of Almond Flour

1 teaspoon of Salt

1/2 cup of Dry Grated Parmesan Cheese

5 Minced Garlic Cloves

1 cup of Chopped Green Pepper

2 tablespoons of Butter

1 tablespoon of Thyme Leaves

1 tablespoon of Chopped Fresh Basil Leaves

1/4 cup of Minced Fresh Parsley Leaves

1/2 teaspoon of Ground Black Pepper

1/4 cup of Heavy Cream

2 teaspoons of Dijon Mustard

2 tablespoons of Ellen's Low-Carb BBQ Sauce

1/2 teaspoon of Unflavored Gelatin

Directions:

1. Preheat your oven to 350 degrees. Grease your 10 x 15 baking dish with your butter. Place to the side.

2. In a small size deep bowl, whisk your Parmesan cheese and almond flour together. Place to the side.

3. Heat your butter in medium skillet over medium heat. Add in garlic, pepper, and onion. Saute till softened. Should be approximately 8 minutes. Place to the side to cool while getting your other ingredients ready. Once your mixture is cool, run it through your food processor to mince your vegetables to a fine consistency.

4. In a separate deep small bowl, whisk your pepper, salt, spices, eggs, BBQ sauce, cream, and mustard. Sprinkle your gelatin over mixture. Let it stand for approximately 5 minutes. Add in your minced onion mixture and mix all together well. Place to the side.

5. Place your ground beef and sausage on a large size cutting board, Mix them together. Make sure no large chunks are left unmixed. Don't knead your meat for more than 5 minutes. If you do it will make your meat tough.

6. Return your low carb meatloaf to a larger size mixing bowl. Add in your egg mix and mix together well. Add in your almond flour mixture. Mix until it is evenly blended together. It should no longer be sticky.

7. Place in your baking dish, making it into a loaf. Leave approximately an inch on all sides. Flatten your loaf shape on top so it all will cook evenly.

8. Bake your meatloaf till browned. Cooking thermometer should read at least 160 degrees. It should take approximately 1 hour. Let it rest for 20 minutes.

9. Serve and Enjoy!

Nutritional Value - (Serving Size 5 Ounces):

23 grams of Protein.

33 grams of Fat.

5 grams of Carbs.

409 Calories.

Spicy Low-Carb Kentucky Stew (Serves 14)

Ingredients:

4 pounds of Pot Roast

28 ounce can of Diced Tomatoes

2 cups of Beef Broth

1 pound of Large Chicken Breast (Shredded and Boiled)

1/4 teaspoon of Thyme

1/4 teaspoon of Celery Salt

2 teaspoon of Dried Dill Weed

1 teaspoon of Basil

1 tablespoon of Garlic Salt

2 teaspoon of Garlic Powder

1 tablespoon of Oregano

2 teaspoon of Pepper

7 ounces of Polish Kielbasa

1 teaspoon of Minced Garlic

1 tablespoon of Powdered Buttermilk

1 1/2 tablespoons of Onion Powder

1 1/2 tablespoons of Dried Parsley

1 cup of Chicken Bone Broth

1 can of Rotel Original

1/2 teaspoon of Red Pepper Flakes

2 teaspoons of Frank's Red Hot Sauce

1/2 medium Chopped Onion

1 tablespoon of Coconut Oil

Directions:

1. Add pot roast and beef broth to your crock pot and set the temperature to low.

2. Combine your dry ingredients in a bowl and rub your pot roast on all sides with them.

3. Cook on low approximately 4 to 8 hours.

4. Boil one large chicken breast for about 40 minutes. Shred once fully cooked. Place in refrigerator.

5. Once pot roast is cook split into half. 2 pounds will go to your stew. Feel free to have other 2 pounds as a separate pot roast meal.

6. Cut roast into cubes and place back in your crockpot.

7. Add in rest of ingredients and cook on low approximately 12 to 24 hours.

8. Flavor to taste with your hot sauce, pepper, and salt.

9. Serve and Enjoy!

Bacon Whiskey Caramelized Onions (Serves 1)

Ingredients:

1 Onion

3 teaspoons of Whiskey

1 tablespoon of Bacon Grease

Water

Directions:

1. Heat pan on medium low with bacon grease.

2. Cut onion in half and then cut into 1/4 inch slices.

3. Add your onions to pan once hot and cook. Use a wooden spoon to break apart onions sticking together.

4. Mix around every couple minutes for approximately 20 minutes.

5. Add a teaspoon of whiskey followed by one teaspoon of water each time onions start getting dry and begin sticking to your pan. Mix well. Be sure to rotate using whiskey and water till all the whiskey is gone.

6. Once onions are soft, brown, and sweet they're done. You don't want onions to get crispy or dry. Make sure not burn.

7. Serve and Enjoy!

Sweet Pea Coconut Hash (Serves 2)

Ingredients:

7 ounces of Stringles Sugar Snap Pea Pods

1/8 teaspoon of Cinnamon

4 tablespoons of Salted Butter

1/2 cup of Unsweetened Shredded Coconut

1 tablespoon of Coconut Oil

1 tablespoon of Rosemary Oil

Salt

Directions:

1. Melt butter in a pan over medium-low heat. Then add in coconut oil.

2. Chop your pea pods into 5 slices per each pea pod.

3. Add your coconut to the pan and then mix until it is fully coated.

4. Add your rosemary oil and cinnamon. Mix until combined.

5. Cook for about 1 minute on low. This will moisten your coconut up.

6. Add your chopped pea pods and mix. Cook for 5 minutes on medium heat.

7. Add a dash of salt.

8. Serve and Enjoy!

Nutritional Value - (Serving Size 1/2):

4.1 grams of Protein.

50.5 grams of Fat.

13.2 grams of Carbs.

509 Calories.

Chapter Nine: Ketogenic Diet Snacks, Drinks, & Condiment Recipes

In this section, I will give you 50 ketogenic snack and condiment recipes you can make yourself. I'll include both basic recipes and a few more advanced recipes. That way no matter what your level in the kitchen you'll be able to prepare healthy low carb keto snacks to keep you on track with your diet. I'll add in the nutritional value whenever possible, although I don't have those exact numbers for every recipe.

Simple Cole Slaw (Serves 16)

Ingredients:

1 head of Green Cabbage

146 grams of Carrots

6 tablespoons of Mayo

60 grams of Green Onion

1 tablespoon of Yellow Mustard

Pepper

Salt

Directions:

1. Peel off the outer layer of your cabbage and discard it.

2. Cut off the head of your cabbage. Cut it in half, then quarter it.

3. Shred your cabbage.

4. Peel carrots then shred them.

5. Combine cabbage, carrots, mayo, pepper, salt, and mustard.

6. Chop green onions and combine with your slaw.

7. Serve and Enjoy!

Nutritional Value - (Serving Size 1/16):

1 gram of Protein.

4 grams of Fat.

6 grams of Carbs.

58 Calories.

Guacamole (Serves 8)

Ingredients:

4 Avocados

1/2 teaspoon of Cayenne Pepper

1 Small Onion

1 tablespoon of Minced Garlic

1 tablespoon of Lime Juice

2 Tomatoes

1 Jalapeno

1/2 teaspoon of Salt

1/2 teaspoon of Cumin

Directions:

1. Peel and chop your avocados.

2. Put in large bowl and toss with your lime juice.

3 Add in spices and mash your avocados.

4. Add your jalapenos, tomatoes, and onions. Mix together well.

5. Store at room temperature for approximately 1 hour.

6. Serve and Enjoy!

Nutritional Value - (Serving Size 1/8):

3 grams of Protein.

11 grams of Fat.

11 grams of Carbs.

140 Calories.

Keto 5 Layer Dip (Serves 10)

Ingredients:

20 ounces of Guacamole

4 ounces of Mayo

4 ounces of Cream Cheese

8 ounces of Sour Cream

16 ounces of Salsa

2 tablespoons of Taco Seasoning

4 ounces of Diced Green Onions

10 ounces of Shredded Cheddar Cheese

Directions:

1. Combine mayo, cream cheese, sour cream, and seasoning.

2. Mix until smooth.

3. Chop green onions.

4. Layer 1 - Use a medium sized casserole dish and spread out guacamole on the bottom.

5. Layer 2 - Carefully spread sour cream mix over top the guacamole.

6. Layer 3 - Spread salsa over your sour cream mixture.

7. Layer 4 - Add your cheese.

8. Layer 5 - Top with your green onions.

9. Refrigerate it between 1 hour and 24 hours.

10. Serve and Enjoy!

Nutritional Value - (Serving Size 1/10):

10 grams of Protein.

29 grams of Fat.

11 grams of Carbs.

343 Calories.

Parmesan Chips (Serves 9)

Ingredients:

4 ounces of Grated Parmesan

4 ounces of Shaved Parmesan

Directions:

1. Preheat your oven to 375 degrees.

2. Layer bottom of your well with grated cheese, followed by shaved cheese, followed by grated cheese.

3. Cook approximately 7 minutes until it is golden brown and crisp.

4. Allow to cool for approximately 5 minutes.

Nutritional Value - (Serving Size 1 Chip):

6 grams of Protein.

3 grams of Fat.

0 grams of Carbs.

60 Calories.

Grilled Avocado (Serves 2)

Ingredients:

2 ounces of Salsa

1 Avocado

Pepper

Salt

Directions:

1. Preheat your grill to a medium-high heat.

2. Slice your avocado in half. Remove and get rid of the pit.

3. Pepper and salt your avocado meat.

4. Put on the grill. Turn every couple minutes until the skin turns greenish and inside has browned.

5. Add a scoop of salsa to center of your avocado.

Nutritional Value - (Serving Size 1/2):

1 gram of Protein.

5 grams of Fat.

5 grams of Carbs.

67 Calories.

Grilled Garlic

Ingredients:

4 Whole Garlic Bulbs

Olive Oil

Pepper

Salt

Directions:

1. Cut tops off your garlic.

2. Soak cloves in ice water approximately 30 minutes.

3. Set grill up for indirect heat. Preheat to 350 degrees.

4. Drain your garlic and put in the center of 12 x 12 square of foil. Have the cut side up.

5. Drizzle garlic with your olive oil. Add your pepper and salt.

6. Fold sides of your foil over to seal it.

7. Grill over the indirect heat approximately 1 hour.

8. Serve and Enjoy!

Roasted Pumpkin Seeds

Ingredients:

Pumpkin Seeds

Seasoning

Oil

Directions:

1. Wash and dry pumpkin seeds.

2. Add oil to bowl with seeds in them. Add your seasoning. Mix well.

3. Line your pan with foil then spread your seeds out.

4. Cook at 400 degrees in the oven, stirring it at 10 minutes and then again 20 minutes, 25 minutes, and 30 minutes.

5. After 30 minutes continue to watch until it's done.

6. Serve and Enjoy!

Nutritional Value - (Serving Size 1/4 Cup):

8 grams of Protein.

15 grams of Fat.

4 grams of Carbs.

180 Calories.

Pesto Spirals (Serves 2)

Ingredients:

1 medium Zucchini

1/2 large Cucumber

5 Radishes

4 tablespoons of Pesto

Directions:

1. Wash your vegetables and cut ends off your zucchini, radishes, and cucumber.

2. Feed them into your spiralizer using the small setting.

3. Turn your vegetable to create your spirals.

4. Cut spirals when at desired length.

5. Add your pesto and mix well.

Nutritional Value - (Serving Size 1/2):

3 grams of Protein.

13 grams of Fat.

9 grams of Carbs.

166 Calories.

Cheesy Pepperoni (Serves 1)

Ingredients:

1 Cheese Stick

7 slices of Pepperoni

Directions:

1. Cook your pepperoni slices in your skillet.

2. Cut your cheese stick in equal parts.

3. Place one of your cheese pieces on one of your pepperoni slices.

4. Serve and Enjoy!

Nutritional Value:

10 grams of Protein.

20 grams of Fat.

0 grams of Carbs.

230 Calories.

Simple Fried Broccoli (Serves 2)

Ingredients:

2 ounces of Bleu Cheese Dressing

1 bunch of Broccoli

1 teaspoon of Frank's Red Hot

Directions:

1. Separate broccoli into florets.

2. Deep fry them until it is crispy and golden brown.

3. Combine hot sauce and bleu cheese as a side dipping sauce.

4. Serve and Enjoy!

Nutritional Value - (Serving Size 1/2):

2 grams of Protein.

17 grams of Fat.

6 grams of Carbs.

177 Calories.

Cheese & Chive Rollups (Serves 9)

Ingredients:

18 Slices of Thin Swiss Cheese

18 Slices of Ham

8-ounce package of Chive and Onion Cream Cheese

Directions:

1. Take out a block of sliced ham and dry off the top slice.

2. Thinly spread out your cream cheese over your ham slices. Use 2 teaspoons per slice.

3. Scrape last 1/2 inch of ham clean.

4. Add a slice of cheese to the 1/2 inch non-scraped side.

5. Starting at cheese side, fold your end of ham over the end of cheese.

6. Tightly roll your ham and cheese up.

7. Slice into small rolls.

8. Serve and Enjoy.

Nutritional Value - (Serving Size 2 Rollups):

18 grams of Protein.

13 grams of Fat.

4 grams of Carbs.

212 Calories.

Deep Fried Jalapeno Poppers (Serves 4)

Ingredients:

Inside:

6 Thick Cut Bacon Slices

1.5 ounces of Jalapeno Slices

4 ounces of Shredded Cheddar Cheese

4 ounces of Cream Cheese

Batter:

2 Eggs

1 tablespoon of Water

2 tablespoons of Parmesan Cheese

4 tablespoons of Almond Flour

Directions:

1. Cook your bacon and crumble it.

2. Chop jalapeno slices.

3. Combine your bacon, cheddar cheese, jalapeno slices, and cream cheese.

4. Form into 20 equal sized balls. Place in refrigerator.

5. Make your batter by whisking your eggs, adding in the Parmesan cheese and almond flour.

6. Coat your balls. Refrigerate again

7. Fry balls until they turn golden brown.

8. Serve and Enjoy!

Nutritional Value - (Serving Size 5 Poppers):

22 grams of Protein.

33 grams of Fat.

4 grams of Carbs.

387 Calories.

Simple Fried Zucchini

Ingredients:

Zucchini

Salt

Directions:

1. Heat fryer to 375 degrees.

2 Wash zucchini then cut off their ends.

3. Slice zucchini thinly into chips or fries. The thinner you make them the better.

4. Fry till they turn golden brown. Turn occasionally when frying.

5. Serve and Enjoy!

Open Faced Quail Egg Sandwich (Serves 3)

Ingredients:

10 Quail Eggs

5 slices of Bacon

2.5 slices of Cheddar Cheese

Pepper

Salt

Standard Almond Bun recipe:

2 Eggs

5 tablespoons of Unsalted Water

1.5 teaspoon of Baking Powder

1.5 teaspoon of Splenda

3/4 cup of Almond Flour

Directions:

1. Mix your almond bun ingredients together. Divide into 10 separate portions on a pie pan.

2. Bake at 350 degrees for 8 to 12 minutes.

3. Cook your bacon.

4. Fry your 10 quail eggs. Top them with pepper and salt.

5. Top each of your almond buns with 1/4 slice of cheese, 1/2 slice of bacon, and one quail egg.

6. Serve and Enjoy!

<u>Nutritional Value (Serving Size 3 1/3 Eggs):</u>

14 grams of Protein.

18 grams of Fat.

1 gram of Carbs.

245 Calories.

Goat Cheese & Zucchini Wraps (Serves 6)

Ingredients:

1 Zucchini

1 teaspoon of Dried Dill

1 teaspoon of Dried Mint

6 ounces of Soft Goat Cheese

Pepper

Salt

Oil

Toothpicks

Directions:

1. Wash zucchini and cut off ends.

2. Using your mandoline, slice your zucchini into 1/8 inch slices.

3. Brush your slices with oil and add pepper and salt.

4. Grill for 5 minutes turning over at the halfway point. Want they to turn brown.

5. Combine your mint, dill, and goat cheese.

6. Dive mixture into 6 servings.

7. Roll goat cheese into cylinder shape between fingers and spread on zucchini.

8. Roll up your zucchini and stick a toothpick through it.

9. Serve and Enjoy!

Nutritional Value - (Serving Size 1 Roll):

13 grams of Protein.

14 grams of Fat.

3 grams of Carbs.

186 Calories.

Deviled Egg Chicks (Serves 10)

Ingredients:

10 Eggs

1 tablespoon of Dijon Mustard

4 tablespoons of Mayo

Carrot Slivers

Dash of Hot Sauce

Olive Slivers

Directions:

1. Place your eggs in your pan and cover with water.

2. Boil eggs for 15 minutes.

3. Shock you eggs with cold water and peel them.

4. Slice eggs in half and separate out your egg yolks.

5. In mixing bowl, combine your mayo, egg yolks, hot sauce, and mustard.

6. Whisk till smooth.

7. Cut bottoms of half the egg halves and middle out rest of them.

8. Pipe in your yolk mix on the bottoms, adding more to the front.

9. Top with rest of egg and add carrot and two olive slices. These will make your nose and eyes.

10. Serve and Enjoy!

Nutritional Value - (Serving Size 1 Egg):

6 grams of Protein.

9 grams of Fat.

0.4 grams of Carbs.

110 Calories.

Bacon Deviled Eggs (Serves 20)

Ingredients:

10 Large Eggs

4 slices of Thick Cut Bacon

5 tablespoons of Mayo

1 tablespoons of Sugar-Free Pickle Relish

Paprika

Directions:

1. Hard boil your eggs.

2. Cover eggs in cold water an inch above them.

3. Apply high heat and once water boils, boil for 15 minutes.

4. Carefully remove water and cover eggs with cold water.

5. Crack eggs all around and roll between hands to peel.

6. Dry your peeled eggs.

7. Cut your eggs lengthwise in half. Separate yolks from your egg whites.

8. In large mixing bowl, crumble your yolks using a fork.

9. Add mayo until your mixture gets a batter consistency.

10. Add your pickle relish and mix well.

11. Add the cooled, crumbled up bacon.

12. Using your fork, fill your egg halves with your yolk mixture.

13. Sprinkle deviled eggs with your paprika.

14. Serve and Enjoy!

Nutritional Value - (Serving Size 1/2 Egg):

4 grams of Protein.

6 grams of Fat.

1 gram of Carbs.

69 Calories.

Mashed Cauliflower (Serves 6)

Ingredients:

1 head of Cauliflower

5 slices of Bacon

2 ounces of Cream Cheese

2 1/2 ounces of Monterey Jack Cheese

2 1/2 ounces of Cheddar Cheese

Pepper

Salt

Directions:

1. Cook your bacon and crumble.

2. Wash, remove leaves and chop your cauliflower.

3. Bring water to boil, add cauliflower and boil approximately 9 minutes.

4. Cube your cheeses while cauliflower boils.

5. Drain your cauliflower.

6. Mash cauliflower, add cream cheese and then mash it again.

7. Season with pepper and salt.

8. Stir in your bacon and cheese. You can stop there or you can also place in a baking dish and bake for 10 minutes at 350 degrees.

9. Serve and Enjoy!

Nutritional Value - (Serving Size 1/6):

12 grams of Protein.

15 grams of Fat.

8 grams of Carbs.

210 Calories.

Garlic Asparagus (Serves 4)

Ingredients:

1 bunch of Asparagus

1 tablespoon of Minced Garlic

2 tablespoons of Butter

Directions:

1. Wash your asparagus then separate your stalks.

2. Boil water and cook asparagus for 2 to 3 minutes.

3. Drain asparagus and then cool down in cold water.

4. Heat your butter and some garlic in your skillet.

5. Fry your asparagus till browning and crisp.

6. Serve and Enjoy!

Nutritional Value - (Serving Size 1/4):

1 gram of Protein.

6 grams of Fat.

3 grams of Carbs.

61 Calories.

Peppery Cheese Biscuits (Serves 37)

Ingredients:

2 Large Eggs

2 1/2 cups of Almond Flour

6 ounces of Shredded Colby Jack Cheese

8 ounces of Cream Cheese

5 tablespoons of Butter

3 teaspoons of Freshly Cracked Black Pepper

1 teaspoon of Baking Soda

3/4 teaspoon of Xanthan Gum

1 teaspoon of Sea Salt

Directions:

1. Preheat your oven to 325 degrees. Line a cookie sheet with your parchment paper.

2. Put 1 cup of almond flour and shredded cheese in food processor. Process until it is finely grained. Put to the side.

3. In glass mixing bowl, place cream cheese and butter. Microwave 30 seconds and remove. Whisk it until it is glossy and smooth.

4. Whisk in your eggs until your mixture is smooth. Mix in baking soda, pepper, salt, and xanthan gum.

5. Add your almond flour cheese mix to egg mixture. Add remaining almond flour and fold in till mixed together well and a dough begins forming.

6. Drop mixture by tablespoon onto cookie sheet. Space each an inch apart. Roll dough a bit to smooth it out so it makes a prettier biscuit.

7. Bake approximately 20 to 25 minutes. Should be golden brown on top. Remove and let it cool down for 10 minutes. Makes approximately 37 biscuits.

8. Serve and Enjoy!

Nutrition Value - (Serving Size 1 roll):

3 grams of Protein.

9 grams of Fat.

2 grams of Carbs.

96 Calories.

Spicy Bacon Cauliflower (Serves 4)

Ingredients:

5 slices of Thick Cut Bacon

16 ounces of Frozen Cauliflower

Old Bay

Directions:

1. Microwave entire bag of cauliflower.

2. Cook your bacon until it is crisp in your oven at 450 degrees.

3. Heat your bacon grease in a skillet.

4. Add your cooked cauliflower to your grease and cover heavily with Old Bay.

5. Saute this for approximately 5 minutes. Be sure to mix around well.

6. Reapply Old Bay.

7. Mix until your cauliflower is well cooked and broken up.

8. Take bacon out of your oven and cut into small pieces. Add it to your mixture.

9. Serve and Enjoy!

Nutritional Value - (Serving Size 1/4):

6 grams of Protein.

6 grams of Fat.

5 grams of Carbs.

100 Calories.

Bacon Brussels Sprouts (Serves 4)

Ingredients:

1/4 cup of Fish Sauce

24 ounces of Brussels Sprouts

1/4 cup of Bacon Grease or Oil

6 strips of Bacon

Pepper

Directions:

1. De-stem and quarter your Brussels sprouts.

2. Mix your Brussels sprouts, fish sauce, and bacon grease.

3. Cook your bacon. Once done cut into smaller strips.

4. Add bacon to your mix and add some pepper. Stir well.

5. On a greased pan spread out your Brussels sprouts.

6. Cook for 40 minutes at 450 degrees, stirring in 10-minute intervals.

7. Finish off your Brussels sprouts on broil for a couple of minutes.

8. Serve and Enjoy!

Nutritional Value - (Serving Size 1/4):

6 grams of Protein.

10 grams of Fat.

8 grams of Carbs.

143 Calories.

Kohlrabi Kraut (Serves 12)

Ingredients:

2 pounds of Ham Hock

4 Shredded Kohlrabi

12 ounces of Salt Pork

1/2 of an Onion

1 teaspoon of Caraway Seeds

1/2 cup of Champagne Vinegar

Directions:

1. Fill a large pot halfway with water and boil on high heat.

2. Add bacon grease to skillet and heat on high.

3. Cut up 1/4 of an onion.

4. Brown your ham hocks in bacon grease.

5. Add your onions to your pan and fry with the ham hocks.

6. Once onions get cooked and ham hocks are browned, add to boiling water and season with pepper and salt.

7. Peel and quarter your kohlrabi.

8. Grate your kohlrabi in your food processor.

9. Grate 1/4 of an onion into your mix.

10. Add your kohlrabi to water and season it with pepper and salt.

11. Add your caraway seeds and champagne vinegar.

12. Cover and let simmer approximately 3 hours. Stir occasionally.

13. If water gets low while simmering add more. The mixture should be covered with water entire 3 hours.

14. Near end of simmer remove ham hocks and separate the bone from the meat. Add meat back into your pot.

15. Serve and Enjoy!

Nutritional Value - (Serving Size 1/12):

14 grams of Protein.

17 grams of Fat.

7 grams of Carbs.

181 Calories.

Bacon Rollups (Serves 1)

Ingredients:

2 slices of Cheddar Cheese

2 slices of Bacon

2 Toothpicks

Directions:

1. Cut each cheese piece vertically into fours.

2. Cook your bacon until it is crisp.

3 Remove bacon and add your cheese quickly.

4. Roll up and skewer roll. Let your bacon crisp and allow your cheese to melt a little bit.

5. Serve and Enjoy!

Nutritional Value - (Serving Size 1):

9 grams of Protein.

12 grams of Fat.

0 grams of Carbs.

135 Calories.

Mashed Rutabagas (Serves 4)

Ingredients:

2 slices of Bacon

400 grams of Peeled and Cubed Rutabagas

8 tablespoons of Sour Cream

4 tablespoons of Butter

4 ounces of Shredded Cheddar Cheese

Directions:

1. Peel and cube rutabaga.

2. Place it in your pan and cover it with water.

3. Boil them and reduce down to a simmer.

4. Fry up two slices of bacon while rutabaga cook.

5. Place rutabagas in your food processor and mix.

6. Add your sour cream, butter, and cheese. Process some more.

7. Fold in your crumbled bacon using a spatula.

8. Serve and Enjoy!

Nutritional Value - (Serving Size 1/4):

11 grams of Protein.

28 grams of Fat.

9 grams of Carbs.

334 Calories.

Cheddar Garlic Biscuits (Serves 37)

Ingredients:

2 Large Eggs

6 ounces of Shredded Colby Jack Cheese

2 1/2 cups of Almond Flour

2 teaspoons of Granulated Garlic

5 tablespoons of Butter

8 ounces of Cream Cheese

1 teaspoon of Sea Salt

1 teaspoon of Baking Soda

3/4 teaspoon of Xanthan Gum

Directions:

1. Preheat your oven to 325 degrees and line your cookie sheet with some parchment paper.

2. In your food processor place shredded cheese and 1 cup of almond flour. Process till finely grained. Put to the side.

3. In glass mixing bowl, place your cream cheese and butter. Microwave for 30 seconds. Whisk till glossy and smooth.

4. Whisk in your eggs until it is smooth. Mix in your baking soda, garlic, salt, and xanthan gum.

5. Add your almond flour cheese mix to egg mixture. Add remaining almond flour and fold in until it is mixed together well and a dough begins forming.

6. Drop mixture by tablespoon onto cookie sheet. Space each an inch apart. Roll dough a bit to smooth it out so it makes a prettier biscuit.

7. Bake approximately 20 to 25 minutes. Should be golden brown on top. Remove and let it cool down for 10 minutes. Makes approximately 37 biscuits.

8. Serve and Enjoy!

Nutritional Value - (Serving Size 1 Roll):

3 grams of Protein.

9 grams of Fat.

2 grams of Carbs.

96 Calories.

Turnip Hash Browns (Serves 2)

Ingredients:

1 Large Egg

1 Rutabaga

2 tablespoons of Bacon Grease

2 ounces of Shredded Cheese

Granulated Garlic

Onion Powder

Pepper

Salt

Directions:

1. Peel and quarter rutabaga. Shred 4 ounces of rutabaga and save the rest for some other recipe.

2. Combine your cheese and egg with rutabaga. Mix Well.

3. Heat your bacon grease in your skillet.

4. Add mixture. Cook for a few minutes turning it once.

5. Serve and Enjoy!

Nutritional Value - (Serving Size 1/2):

8 grams of Protein.

20 grams of Fat.

6 grams of Carbs.

231 Calories.

Kale & Bacon Chips

Ingredients:

1 bunch of Kale

1/4 cup of Bacon Grease

2 tablespoons of Butter

2 teaspoons of Salt

Garlic Powder

Directions:

1. Preheat your oven to approximately 300 degrees. Line your cookie sheet with some parchment paper.

2. Remove leaves from kale. Tear kale into smaller bit sized pieces. Wash and dry thoroughly.

3. Add your butter to bacon grease and warm till in a liquid state. Add in your salt and stir.

4. Put kale in a gallon sized Ziploc bag. Add your liquid butter and bacon grease mixture. Don't completely seal bag. You have to be able to shake kale leaves around so they can get completely coated. You want the leaves shiny green. No dry leaves.

5. Pour bag onto your cookie sheet. Make sure leaves are all in a single layer and completely coated. Sprinkle with your garlic powder.

6. Bake approximately 20 to 25 minutes till leaves turn dark green and get crispy but not burnt.

7. Serve and Enjoy.

Nutritional Value - (Serving Size 1 Cup Cooked):

1 gram of Protein.

6 grams of Fat.

1 gram of Carbs.

62 Calories.

Sauteed Cauliflower

Ingredients:

1 tablespoon of Bacon Grease

255 grams of Cauliflower

Pepper

Salt

Directions:

1. Boil your cauliflower for approximately 5 to 10 minutes.

2. Squeeze any liquid out of your cauliflower using a potato ricer.

3. Fry it in your bacon grease. Season when nearly finished cooking.

4. Serve and Enjoy!

Sauteed Mushrooms (Serves 2)

Ingredients:

3 tablespoons of Bacon Grease

10 ounces of White Button Mushrooms

1 teaspoon of Parmesan Cheese

Garlic

Pepper

Salt

Directions:

1. Slice your mushrooms.

2. Cook mushrooms with bacon grease in a skillet.

3. Season with garlic powder, pepper, and salt.

4. Grate Parmesan cheese onto your mushrooms.

Nutritional Value - (Serving Size 1/2)

4 grams of Protein.

17 grams of Fat.

4 grams of Carbs.

185 Calories.

Bacon Wrapped Smokies

Ingredients:

40 to 45 Smokies / Cocktail Wieners

10 slices of Bacon

40 to 45 Toothpicks

Directions:

1. Cut your bacon into 3 or 4 strips.

2. Wrap each of your wieners with a slice of bacon and spear it with one toothpick.

3. Cook at 400 degrees till done. Finish them off with your broiler.

Bacon Wrapped Asparagus

Ingredients:

8 slices of Bacon

40 spears of Asparagus

Directions:

1. Wash your asparagus.

2. Bend each asparagus and break at a weak point. Throw out the base part.

3. Make a bundle of 5 asparagus spears and wrap with one piece of bacon.

4. Bake it at 400 degrees until it is done. Finish them off with your broiler.

Coffee Smoothie (Serves 2)

Ingredients:

6 ounces of Cold Coffee

4 ounces of Heavy Cream

4 ounces of Unsweetened Milk

1 ounce of Torani Sugar-Free Caramel Syrup

1 ounce of Torani Sugar-Free Chocolate Syrup

2 tablespoons of Unsweetened Cocoa

16 ounces of Ice

Directions:

1. Add your liquids to your blender, then add your powder and finally your ice.

2. Use smoothie setting on Vitamix with your tamper attachment to push your mix towards blades.

Nutritional Value - (Serving Size 16 Ounces):

3 grams of Protein.

22 grams of Fat.

6 grams of Carbs.

216 Calories.

Avocado Shake (Serves 1)

Ingredients:

3 ounces of Heavy Whipping Cream

3 ounces of Unsweetened Almond Milk

1 Avocado

6 drops of EZ-Sweetz

6 Ice Cubes

Directions:

1. Add almond milk, EZ-Sweetz, and heavy whipping cream to your Vitamix.

2. Cut your avocado in half and remove seed. Remove flesh from skin and add to your mixer.

3. Add in 6 ice cubes.

4. Blend on your smoothie setting. For regular blender keep blending till mixture has a yogurt consistency.

5. Serve and Enjoy!

Nutritional Value:

6 grams of Protein.

58 grams of Fat.

18 grams of Carbs.

587 Calories.

Raspberry Lemonade Poptail (Serves 2)

Ingredients:

60 milliliters of Heavy Cream

10 milliliters of Lemon Juice

25 milliliters of Torani Sugar-Free Raspberry Syrup

5 milliliters of Vanilla

20 milliliters of Vodka

Directions:

1. Freeze your Zoku device 24 hours till fully frozen.

2. Each popsicle uses 60 milliliters of your total mix.

3. Mix your ingredients and then place in your freezer.

4. Bring out your Zoku device and place your popsicle stick into it.

5. Add your liquid and wait for approximately 16 minutes. May take a little longer to freeze due to the alcohol in it.

6. Once completely frozen, screw on your extractor and release from the mold.

7. Snap your drip shield on.

8. Serve and Enjoy!

Nutritional Value - (Serving Size 1 Popsicle):

0 grams of Protein.

10 grams of Fat.

1 grams of Carbs.

125 Calories.

White Russian Poptail (Serves 2)

Ingredients:

20 milliliters of Unsweetened Coconut Milk

60 milliliters of Heavy Cream

20 milliliters of Da Vinci Sugar-Free Kahlua Syrup

20 milliliters of Vodka

Directions:

1. Freeze your Zoku device 24 hours till fully frozen.

2. Each popsicle uses 60 milliliters of your total mix.

3. Mix your ingredients and then place in your freezer.

4. Bring out your Zoku device and place your popsicle stick into it.

5. Add your liquid and wait for approximately 16 minutes. May take a little longer to freeze due to the alcohol in it.

6. Once completely frozen, screw on your extractor and release from the mold.

7. Snap your drip shield on.

8. Serve and Enjoy!

Nutritional Value - (Serving Size 1 Popsicle):

0 grams of Protein.

10 grams of Fat.

1 gram of Carbs.

125 Calories.

Whipped Eggnog (Serves 4)

Ingredients:

3/4 cup of Heavy Cream

2 Egg Yolks

18 drops of EZ-Sweetz

1/4 cup of Bourbon

Ground Nutmeg

Directions:

1. Mix your ingredients in your bowl.

2. I use an iSi Mini Whip to make my whip cream. Charge up the charger and add it to your canister.

3. Pressurize it with Nitrogen.

4. Shake it 3 to 4 times.

5. Pour into a bowl.

5. Dust with nutmeg.

6. Serve and Enjoy!

Nutritional Value - (Serving Size 1/4):

1 gram of Protein.

17 grams of Fat.

0 grams of Carbs.

212 Calories.

Alcohol-Infused Whipped Cream (Serves 10)

Ingredients:

200 milliliters of Heavy Cream

50 milliliters of Vanilla Vodka

1/4 teaspoon of EZ-Sweetz

1/4 teaspoon of Vanilla

Directions:

1. Combine all your ingredients and place in your iSi Mini Easy Whip Container.

2. Charge it with a Nitrogen cartridge.

3. Shake 3 to 4 times, if it comes out a little runny just shake some more.

4. Pour into a bowl or on top of drink or dessert.

5. Serve and Enjoy.

Nutritional Value - (Serving Size 1/10):

0 grams of Protein.

1 gram of Fat.

0 grams of Carbs.

23 Calories.

Keto Margaritas

Ingredients:

1.5 ounces of Tequila

1 Lime

4 drops of Sucralose

Directions:

1. Cut your lime in half and squeeze it into your container.

2. Fill an old fashion glass with regular ice or crushed ice.

3. Measure 1.5 ounces of lime juice into your glass.

4. Measure 1.5 ounces of tequila into your glass.

5. Add 4 drops of sucralose.

6. Mix and then garnish with a lime slice.

7. Serve and Enjoy!

Keto Apple Martini (Serves 1)

Ingredients:

2 ounces of Plain Vodka

2 ounces of Apple Flavored Vodka

1 teaspoon of Low-Carb Sugar Syrup

Apple slice

Directions:

1. Finely dice your apple slice and place it in your cocktail shaker.

2. Add your sugar syrup and then mash them both together.

3. Add both types of your vodka and ice. Shake it well.

4. Strain it into your martini glass.

5. Serve and Enjoy!

Blueberry Martini (Serves 1)

Ingredients:

2 ounces of Plain Vodka

2 ounces of Blueberry Flavored Vodka

6 or 7 Fresh Blueberries

1 teaspoon of Low-Carb Sugar Syrup

Directions:

1. Place your blueberries in your cocktail shaker.

2. Add your sugar syrup and then mash them both together.

3. Add both types of your vodka and ice. Shake it well.

4. Strain it into your martini glass.

5. Serve and Enjoy!

Low-Carb Keto Mojito (Serves 1)

Ingredients:

2 1/2 ounces of Light Rum

7 to 8 Mint Leaves w/ Stems

1 Lime

1 tablespoon of Low-Carb Sugar Syrup

Club Soda

Directions:

1. Finely dice your mint leaves and mix with your sugar syrup using a tall glass.

2. Cut your lime in half. Discard seeds. Squeeze juice from both halves into your glass.

3. Add your rum and stir.

4. Add your ice and club soda.

5. Serve and Enjoy!

Low-Carb Keto Pina Colada (Serves 2)

Ingredients:

3 ounces of Rum

2/3 cup of Sugar-Free Cream or Coconut Milk

1/2 cup of Sugar-Free Pineapple Syrup

2 cups of Crushed Ice

Directions

1. Add your ingredients to your blender and mix until they get slushy.

2. Pour equally into two glasses.

3. Serve and Enjoy!

Keto Raspberry Vinaigrette

Ingredients:

1/2 cup of White Wine Vinegar

1/2 cup of Golden Raspberries

1/2 cup of Extra Virgin Olive Oil

35 drops of Liquid Stevia

Directions:

1. Combine your olive oil, vinegar, and liquid Stevia into a container that you can fit in an immersion blender.

2. Add your raspberries to a container and blend it well using the immersion blender.

3. Strain your seeds out from vinaigrette, saving the liquid portion. Pour on top of your salad.

4. Serve and Enjoy!

Nutritional Value - (Serving Size 2 Tablespoons):

0.1 grams of Protein.

9.3 grams of Fat.

0.3 grams of Carbs.

84 Calories.

Simple Bleu Cheese Dressing (Serves 2)

Ingredients:

2 ounces of Mayo

3 ounces of Bleu Cheese

1 ounce of Sour Cream

1/2 tablespoon of Lemon Juice

1 ounce of Cream Cheese

Directions:

1. Add your 2 ounces of bleu cheese and rest of your ingredients into your immersion blender.

2. Run blender till finely grated.

3. Once you've blended it, crumble in your remaining 1 ounce of bleu cheese.

4. Serve and Enjoy!

Nutritional Value - (Serving Size 1/2):

12 grams of Protein.

38 grams of Fat.

2 grams of Carbs.

401 Calories.

Keto Blackberry Chipotle Jam (Serves 10)

Ingredients:

8 ounces of Blackberries

8 drops of Liquid Stevia

1 1/2 Chipotle in Adobo

1/4 cup of MCT Oil

1/4 cup of Erythritol

1/4 teaspoon of Guar Gum

Directions:

1. Add your blackberries to your pan over a low heat. Allow it to cook slightly so it becomes soft. Cook approximately 5 minutes.

2. Add your chipotle in adobo to your mixture.

3. Add your erythritol and the Stevia to your pan and mix into blackberries. Crush your blackberries using a fork and mix together.

4. Add your MCT Oil to your pan and turn the heat to medium. Allow your jam to boil, reduce the heat to low and allow to simmer for 6 to 8 minutes.

5. Add your guar gum to jam and mix well. Continue to mix it for approximately 1 to 2 minutes till mixture thickens.

6. Strain your seeds from jam using colander and back of metal spoon. Discard the seeds when done.

7. Serve and Enjoy!

Nutritional Value - (Serving Size 1/10):

0.3 grams of Protein.

5.7 grams of Fat.

1.1 grams of Carbs.

51 Calories.

Horseradish Sauce (Serves 8)

Ingredients:

1/4 cup of Sour Cream

1 teaspoon of Dijon Mustard

3/4 tablespoon of Prepared Horseradish

1 tablespoon of Mayo

Directions:

1. Mix your ingredients together and then serve cold.

Nutritional Value - (Serving Size 1/8):

0 grams of Protein.

3 grams of Fat.

1 grams of Carbs.

30 Calories.

Keto Caesar Dressing (Serves 8)

Ingredients:

3 cloves of Minced Garlic

1 1/2 teaspoons of Anchovy Paste

1 1/2 teaspoons of Dijon Mustard

2 tablespoons of Fresh Lemon Juice

3/4 cup of Mayo

1 teaspoon of Worcestershire Sauce

Pepper

Salt

Directions:

1. Mince your garlic cloves and use a garlic press. Add to large bowl.

2. Add your anchovy paste, lemon juice, Worcestershire sauce, and Dijon mustard to your garlic and whisk it all together.

3. Add your mayonnaise to bowl and whisk till it's all combined.

4. Serve and Enjoy!

Nutritional Value - (Serving Size 2 Tablespoons):

0.1 grams of Protein.

15.1 grams of Fat.

0.8 grams of Carbs.

140 Calories.

Simple Cheese Dip (Serves 12)

Ingredients:

2 pounds of Extra Sharp Cheddar

16 ounces of Mayo

1 Small Onion

8 dashes of Frank's Red Hot

1 tablespoon of Worcestershire Sauce

3 tablespoons of Lemon Juice

Directions:

1. Shred your cheddar cheese and place it in a big mixing bowl.

2. Shred your onions and add it to bowl.

3. Add in all your other ingredients.

4. Mix together well.

Nutritional Value - (Serving Size 1/12):

19 grams of Protein.

51 grams of Fat.

2 grams of Carbs.

540 Calories.

Keto Pesto (Serves 1)

Ingredients:

3/4 cup of Parmesan

1 1/2 cups of Basil

1/3 cup of Toasted Pine Nuts

2/3 cup of Olive Oil

2 teaspoons of Tomato Paste

1 teaspoon of Minced Garlic

Pepper

Salt

Directions:

1. Add your fresh basil to a container.

2. Add your toasted pine nuts to the same container. Toast in a pan over low heat if you did not get them already toasted.

3. Add rest of your ingredients, except your oil and use your immersion blender to help blend everything all together. Add oil slowly as blending.

4. Serve and Enjoy!

Nutritional Value - (Serving Size 1 Tablespoon):

1.3 grams of Protein.

8.9 grams of Fat.

0.4 grams of Carbs.

84 Calories.

Chapter Ten: Ketogenic Diet Dessert Recipes

In this section, I will give you 50 ketogenic dessert recipes you can make yourself. I'll include both basic recipes and a few more advanced recipes. That way no matter what your level in the kitchen you'll be able to prepare healthy low carb keto treats to keep you on track with your diet. I'll add in the nutritional value whenever possible, although I don't have those exact numbers for every recipe.

Almond Joy Fat Bombs (Serves 15)

Ingredients:

1/4 cup of Shredded Coconut

1/2 of Low-Carb Chocolate Bar

15 Almonds

1 tablespoon of Erythritol

1 tablespoon of Coconut Oil

Heart Shaped Candy Mold

Directions:

1. Melt your chocolate bar. Pour half a teaspoon of your melted chocolate bar into candy mold and add an almond to each.

2. Freeze and start working on next step.

3. Combine shredded coconut and your coconut oil. Then add your erythritol and combine together.

4. Add a teaspoon of coconut mixture to candy molds and gently press to create a flat layer on top.

5. Freeze for another 5 minutes so coconut oil solidifies.

6. Finish your candies off using rest of your chocolate mixture and then smooth out the top of candy mold.

7. Freeze for at least 1 hour.

8. Pop out your candies.

9. Serve and Enjoy!

Nutritional Value - (Serving Size 1 Almond Joy Fat Bomb):

0.5 grams of Protein.

4.7 grams of Fat.

0.5 grams of Carbs.

50 Calories.

Pumpkin Pie Fat Bombs (Serves 15)

Ingredients:

2 ounces of Coconut Butter

1/2 cup of Pumpkin Puree

1/4 cup of Erythritol

1/2 cup of Chopped Pecans

2 teaspoons of Pumpkin Pie Spice

1/2 cup of Coconut Oil

Directions:

1. Melt your coconut oil if not already a liquid. Melt coconut butter so it's soft and easy to work with.

2. Combine your coconut butter, coconut oil, and pumpkin puree in mixing bowl. Stir well till all combined together.

3. Add your erythritol.

4. Add your pumpkin pie spice.

5. Add your batter mixture to candy molds, ice cube trays, or containers.

6. Toast some of your chopped pecans over medium heat in a dry pan till fragrant and slightly browned.

7. Top each of your fat bombs with pecan pieces and press them in gently so they stick.

8. Refrigerate until they all set.

9. Serve and Enjoy!

Nutritional Value - (Serving Size 1/15):

1 gram of Protein.

12 grams of Fat.

1 gram of Carbs.

125 Calories.

White Chocolate Butter Pecan Fat Bombs (Serves 4)

Ingredients:

2 ounces of Cocoa Butter

2 tablespoons of Coconut Oil

2 tablespoons of Butter

1 pinch of Salt

1 pinch of Stevia

2 tablespoons of Powdered Erythritol

1/2 cup of Chopped Pecans

1/4 teaspoon of Vanilla Extract

Directions:

1. Melt your butter, coconut butter, and coconut oil together in a pan until it is melted. Turn off heat.

2. Add powdered erythritol to butter mixture and stir well.

3. Add a pinch of salt, Stevia, and vanilla extract.

4. Add some chopped pecans to your silicone cupcake molds or candy molds.

5. Pour your white chocolate mix into your molds evenly and place them in the freezer.

6. Freeze approximately 30 minutes.

7. Serve and Enjoy!

Nutritional Value - (Serving Size 1 Fat Bomb):

0.7 grams of Protein.

30 grams of Fat.

0.25 grams of Carbs.

87 Calories.

Coconut Butter Cup Fat Bombs (Serves 4)

Ingredients:

4 tablespoons of Cocoa Powder

4 tablespoons of Coconut Oil

4 teaspoons of Coconut Butter

2 tablespoons of Erythritol

1 pinch of Salt

Directions:

1. Combine your cocoa powder, erythritol, and coconut oil. Stir till no clumps are left. Add a pinch of salt.

2. Warm up coconut butter if not soft enough.

3. Pour half your chocolate mixture into 4 silicone cupcake molds evenly. Tilt each mold so the chocolate will coat the edge a bit. Place in your freezer for approximately 5 minutes.

4. When this has hardened, spoon a teaspoon of your coconut butter into each of your molds. Spread them evenly on each mold so it covers entire chocolate layer. Place in freezer for approximately 5 minutes.

5. Take your remaining half of chocolate mix and use to cover the hardened coconut butter layer. Spread evenly. Freeze again for approximately 5 minutes.

6. Serve and Enjoy!

Nutritional Value - (Serving Size 1 Fat Bomb):

3 grams of Protein.

26 grams of Fat.

0.5 grams of Carbs.

260 Calories.

Chocolate Chia Pudding - (2 Servings)

Ingredients:

3 tablespoons of Chia Seeds.

1 scoop of Chocolate Protein Powder or Cocoa Powder

1/4 cup of Fresh or Frozen Raspberries

1 cup of Unsweetened Almond Milk or Skim Milk

1 teaspoon of Honey - Only if not using the Protein Powder

Directions:

1. Mix your chocolate protein powder and almond milk together. Make sure you've stirred it well.

2. Add in your Chia Seeds. Make sure you've stirred it in well.

3. Let your mix rest for approximately 5 minutes and then stir.

4. Stir again approximately 5 minutes later.

5. Let mix rest for about 30 minutes in your refrigerator.

6. Add your raspberries on the top.

7. Serve and Enjoy!

Nutritional Value - (Serving Size 1/2):

30 grams of Protein.

12 grams of Fat.

19 grams of Carbs.

235 Calories.

Chocolate Strawberry Mousse (Serves 1)

Ingredients:

1 Strawberry

1/3 cup of Heavy Whipping Cream

4 Drops of EZ-Sweet

2.5 grams of Unsweetened Cocoa

1/2 Scoop of Chocolate Whey Powder

Flakes of 90% Chocolate

Directions:

1, Measure your cream into a container.

2. Add your EZ-Sweet.

3. Add your strawberry.

4. Add your powder.

5. Add your chocolate flakes.

6. Mix 1 to 2 minutes till stiff.

7. Serve and Enjoy!

Nutritional Value:

10 grams of Protein.

33 grams of Fat.

12 grams of Carbs.

330 Calories.

Mexican Chocolate Pudding (Serves 2)

Ingredients:

1 tablespoon of Coconut Milk

1 Avocado

2 1/2 tablespoons of Raw Cocoa Powder

1 teaspoon of Ceylon Cinnamon

1/16 teaspoon of Ground Cayenne Pepper

1 tablespoon of Coconut Milk

1 tablespoon of Sweetener

1/2 teaspoon of Pure Vanilla Extract

1 pinch of Pink Himalayan Sea Salt

1 pinch of Stevia

Directions:

1. Cut and pit your avocado. Blend in food processor till smooth.

2. Add your coconut milk, vanilla extract, and cocoa powder. Blend it until it is smooth.

3. Add your cinnamon, sweetener, ground cayenne pepper, and Stevia.

4. Blend till smooth. Get rid of all chunks.

5. Sprinkle with sea salt.

6. Serve and Enjoy!

Nutritional Value - (Serving Size 1/2):

3 grams of Protein.

15 grams of Fat.

3.5 grams of Carbs.

180 Calories.

Peanut Butter Cookies (Serves 15)

Ingredients:

1 Egg

1/2 cup of Powdered Erythritol

1 cup of Peanut Butter

Directions:

1. Preheat oven to 350 degrees.

2. Combine ingredients and mix well.

3. Roll your mix into 1-inch balls and place on a baking sheet lined with parchment paper.

4. Bake approximately 10 to 15 minutes till cookie edges begin to turn dark brown.

5. Allow to cool on wire rack.

6. Serve and Enjoy!

Nutritional Value - (Serving Size 1 Cookie):

4 grams of Protein.

9 grams of Fat.

2 grams of Carbs.

105 Calories.

Quest Cookies (Serves 1)

Ingredients:

1 Quest Bar

Directions:

1. Preheat oven to 450 degrees.

2. Microwave bar for 10 seconds.

3. Break into 8 evenly sized parts and roll up into balls.

4. Put on your baking sheet and cook approximately 3 minutes.

5. Serve and Enjoy!

Nutritional Value:

21 grams of Protein.

8 grams of Fat.

20 grams of Carbs.

190 Calories.

Cake Batter Cookies (Serves 12)

Ingredients:

Cookies

1/4 cup of Softened Butter

1 Egg

1 cup of Sukrin Gold

1/4 cup of Erythritol

1 Egg Yolk

1 teaspoon of Vanilla Extract

1 1/2 teaspoons of Butter Extract

1/4 teaspoon of Almond Extract

3/4 cup of Almond Flour

1/2 teaspoon of Salt

1 tablespoon of Coconut Flour

2 tablespoons of Rainbow Sprinkles

1/2 teaspoon of Xanthan Gum

Optional Filling

1/4 cup of Softened butter

1/2 cup of Sukrin Melis

Directions:

1. Cream together your erythritol, Sukrin Gold, and softened butter with electric hand mixer.

2. Mix in egg yolk and egg.

3. Add butter, almond, and vanilla extracts.

4. Add your salt and flours. Mix it well until it is combined.

5. Add your xanthan gum. Mix until your batter thickens.

6. Mix in sprinkles and stir to evenly distribute them.

7. Refrigerate batter for a little bit.

8. Lay out saran wrap and place cookie batter onto it.

9. Wrap your batter into log 3-inches thick. Make sure the thickness is uniform throughout. Refrigerate 2 hours to allow to harden.

10. Take out of your refrigerator and preheat your oven to 350 degrees. Unwrap your log and roll to get rid of flattened edges. Slice log into desired cookie thickness. For this example, I cut them into 12 cookies.

11. Line cookies on baking sheet lined with parchment paper and cook approximately 10 minutes. Cookies are done when slightly golden.

12. Allow cookies to cool down.

13. You can make the optional filling above combining two ingredients. Then put on top of a cookie and place another cookie on top making into a cookie sandwich.

14. Serve and Enjoy!

Nutritional Value - (Serving Size 1 Cookie):

3 grams of Protein.

17 grams of Fat.

2 grams of Carbs.

175 Calories.

Blueberry Lemon Shortbread Cookies (Serves 9)

Ingredients:

Cookies

1 Egg

1/2 cup of Sukrin Sweetener

1/4 cup of Softened Butter

1 Egg Yolk

1 teaspoon of Vanilla Extract

1 tablespoon of Lemon Juice

3/4 cup of Sifted Almond Flour

1/2 teaspoon of Salt

1/2 teaspoon of Baking Powder

1/2 teaspoon of Xanthan Gum

1 tablespoon of Coconut Flour

Blueberry Glaze

1/4 cup of Blueberries

1/4 cup of Coconut Oil

2 tablespoons of Sukrin Melis

Directions:

1. Preheat oven to 350 degrees.

2. Beat together your butter and Sukrin until it is creamy.

3. Add in egg yolk and egg along with your vanilla and lemon juice. Mix it well.

4. In a different bowl, sift almond flour and combine with rest of dry ingredients excluding your xanthan gum.

5. Slowly pour dry ingredients into wet ingredients, beating your mixture the entire time.

6. When all combined add your xanthan gum and mix it well.

7. Line your baking sheet using parchment paper and measure out evenly sized cookie dough balls. Flatten each one and ensure each one cooks evenly.

8. Bake approximately 8 to 10 minutes.

9. Allow to cool completely.

10. Make your glaze. Combine all ingredients in your immersion blender or Nutribullet.

11. Allow glaze to sit and thicken up. Put a teaspoon of glaze over each of your cookies.

12. Refrigerate glazed cookies for an hour.

13. Serve and Enjoy!

Nutritional Value - (Serving Size 1 Cookie):

3 grams of Protein.

17 grams of Fat.

2 grams of Carbs.

170 Calories.

Keto Mug Cookie (Serves 1)

Ingredients:

1 Egg Yolk

1 tablespoon of Butter

1 tablespoon of Erythritol

3 tablespoons of Almond Flour

1 pinch of Cinnamon

1 pinch of Salt

2 tablespoons of Sugar-Free Chocolate Chips

1/8 teaspoon of Vanilla Extract

Directions:

1. Preheat oven to 350 degrees.

2. Melt butter in small pan and allow to brown a bit.

3. Combine butter with almond flour.

4. Add in cinnamon and erythritol.

5. Add your vanilla extract, egg yolk, and salt.

6. Spray cup or mug with cooking oil and place in your mixture. Flatten it out to make sure it cooks evenly.

7. Press into your cup.

8. Microwave for 1 minute on high or bake in your oven approximately 10 minutes.

9. Allow to cool.

10. Serve and Enjoy!

Nutritional Value:

7 grams of Protein.

31 grams of Fat.

3 grams of Carbs.

330 Calories.

Cinnamon Coconut Peanut Butter Cookies (Serves 15)

Ingredients:

1 Egg

1 cup of Peanut Butter

1/2 cup of Erythritol

1/4 cup of Butter

1 tablespoon of Cinnamon

2 tablespoons of Shredded Coconut

1/2 teaspoon of Vanilla Extract

1 pinch of Salt

Directions:

1. Preheat your oven to 350 degrees. Beat together your butter, peanut butter, erythritol, and egg.

2. Add in cinnamon, shredded coconut, salt and fold it all in together.

3. Roll into balls about 1 1/2 inches in diameter. Lay out on a baking sheet lined with parchment paper.

4. Sprinkle with shredded coconut.

5. Bake approximately 15 minutes. Edges should become golden colored.

6. Allow to cool.

7. Serve and Enjoy!

<u>Nutritional Value - (Serving Size 1 Cookie):</u>

4 grams of Protein.

12 grams of Fat.

2 grams of Carbs.

140 Calories.

Coconut Macaroons (Serves 10)

Ingredients:

4 Egg Whites

1 teaspoon of Vanilla

½ teaspoon of EZ-Sweet

4 1/2 teaspoons of Water

2 cups of Unsweetened Coconut

Directions:

1. Combine egg whites and liquids.

2. Add in coconut and mix together.

3. Spread on your greased pie pan.

4. Preheat oven to 375 degrees. When you put in your macaroons reduce heat to 325 degrees and bake for approximately 14 minutes.

Nutritional Value - (Serving Size 1 Cookie)

2 grams of Protein.

8 grams of Fat.

3 grams of Carbs.

88 Calories.

Keto Ice Cream (Serves 4)

Ingredients:

1/2 cup of Heavy Cream

16 drops of EZ-Sweetz

1 tablespoon of Lemon Juice

3 ounces of Cream Cheese

8 Strawberries

1/4 teaspoon of Vanilla Extract

3/4 cup of Ice

Directions:

1. Place ingredients in your Vitamix.

2. Using the variable speed setting, start on 1 till solids are pulverized then rotate to 10 slowly while you use your tamper to push ingredients into blades. Blend together for 30 to 60 seconds until mounds begin to form.

3. Serve and Enjoy!

Nutritional Value - (Serving Size 1/4):

4 grams of Protein.

16 grams of Fat.

5 grams of Carbs.

179 Calories.

Butter Pecan Ice Cream (Serves 6)

Ingredients:

2 Egg Yolks

1 cup of Heavy Cream

2 tablespoons of Butter

1 teaspoon of Vanilla Extract

1/3 cup of Erythritol

2/3 cups of Chopped Pecans

1 pinch of Stevia

1/8 teaspoon of Xanthan Gum

Directions:

1. Melt butter in your pan over a low flame. Allow to brown slightly.

2. Add in your cream and let it simmer.

3. Turn heat to lowest setting, adding your erythritol. Allow to completely dissolve. Stir gently.

4. Transfer your mixture into a large mixing bowl. Add Stevia. Use your electric hand mixer to get your ingredients combined.

5. While mixing on the medium setting, add your xanthan gum to allow your ingredients to thicken and bind.

6. In another small bowl, separate your egg yolks and add in your vanilla extract. Slowly beat them into your mixing bowl as you're beating the cream mixture.

7. Add chopped pecans and fold in using a spoon.

8. Place bowl in your freezer. Take out to stir every 40 minutes so pecans are well incorporated.

9. Allow to freeze for at least 3 hours before serving.

10. Serve and Enjoy!

Nutritional Value - (Serving Size 1/6):

2 grams of Protein.

20 grams of Fat.

1 gram of Carbs.

200 Calories.

Strawberry Swirl Ice Cream (Serves 6)

Ingredients:

3 large Egg Yolks

1 cup of Heavy Cream

1/3 cup of Erythritol

1/2 teaspoon of Vanilla Extract

1 cup of Pureed Strawberries

1/8 teaspoon of Xanthan Gum (optional)

1 tablespoon of Vodka (optional)

Directions:

1. Set a pot with your heavy cream over a low flame to heat up. Add in your erythritol.

2. Don't let the cream boil, just let it gently simmer till the erythritol is all dissolved.

3. Separate your egg yolks into a large mixing bowl. Beat with your electric mixer until doubled in size.

4. Temper eggs so they don't scramble, add a couple tablespoons of the heated cream mixture at a time to the eggs while you're beating them.

5. Continue until your egg mixture is warm and then add in the rest of your cream mixture slowly, beating them constantly.

6. Add in your vanilla extract and mix.

7. Optional step. Add in vodka and xanthan gum.

8. Place bowl in freezer and leave for 2 hours occasionally taking out to stir, Can also churn using your ice cream maker if you have one.

9. Puree your strawberries. I use my Nutribullet.

10. Once the ice cream has been chilled and is beginning to thicken add in your pureed strawberries.

11. Mix in strawberries but don't mix too much. You want ribbons of your strawberry visible in the ice cream.

12. Place in freezer for 4 to 6 hours.

13. Serve and Enjoy!

Nutritional Value - (Serving Size 1/6):

2.3 grams of Protein.

16.9 grams of Fat.

2.8 grams of Carbs.

178 Calories.

Mint Chocolate Chip Ice Cream (Serves 4)

Ingredients:

1 cup of Heavy Cream

1/2 cup of Light Cream

1/2 teaspoon of Liquid Stevia Extract

1/2 teaspoon of Vanilla (Optional)

1 Square Dark Chocolate (Optional)

Several drops of Green Food Coloring (Optional)

Several drops of Peppermint Extract (Optional)

Directions:

1. Place ice cream bowl in your freezer 4 to 12 hours ahead of time.

2. Place all ingredients in ice cream bowl except the chocolate.

3. Whisk together well.

4. Place in your freezer for approximately 5 minutes.

5. Set up your ice cream maker and add in liquid.

6. Make ice cream according to your machine's instructions. A few minutes before ice cream sets, add in your chocolate shavings.

7. Store in air tight container and place back in the freezer.

8. Allow to freeze.

9. Serve and Enjoy!

Nutritional Value - (Serving Size 1/4):

2.25 grams of Protein.

31 grams of Fat.

3.5 grams of Carbs.

295 Calories.

Chocolate Chip Peanut Butter Ice Cream

Ingredients:

3 large Egg Yolks

1/2 cup of Almond Milk

1/2 cup of Heavy Cream

1/4 cup of Erythritol

1/2 cup of Peanut Butter

1/4 teaspoon of Xanthan Gum

1 teaspoon of Vanilla Extract

3/4 cup of Sugar-Free Chocolate Chips

1 tablespoon of Vodka (Optional)

Directions:

1. Heat erythritol and heavy cream on a stove over a low heat. Don't boil. Let it come to a gentle simmer.

2. While that's heating up, whisk together egg yolks and add in your vanilla extract.

3. Temper eggs so they don't scramble by slowly adding hot cream while continuing to whisk.

4. Pour tempered eggs into your hot cream and whisk over a low flame.

5. Add in xanthan gum and mix till everything thickens up.

6. Transfer to your bowl and add vodka if you're using it. Chill until it is cooled down.

7. Once your mixture is cool, add to your ice cream maker and follow the instructions for that machine.

8. Once ice cream is thick in your ice cream maker, add your chocolate chips. In last few seconds of churning, add in your peanut butter.

9. Place in your freezer if you want it harder.

10. Serve and Enjoy!

Nutritional Value - (Serving Size 1/2 Cup):

8 grams of Protein.

26 grams of Fat.

5.8 grams of Carbs.

295 Calories.

Keto Popsicles (Serves 2)

Ingredients:

4 tablespoons of Heavy Cream

4 teaspoons of Sugar-Free Flavored Syrup

2 1/3 tablespoons of Sugar-Free Coconut Milk

Directions:

1. Freeze your Zoku device at for approximately 1 day or until completely frozen.

2. Each popsicle will use 4 tablespoons of your total mix. Mix ingredients and put in the freezer.

3. Bring out your Zoku and place a popsicle stick in it.

4. Add your liquid and wait approximately 9 minutes.

5. Once completely frozen, screw in your extractor and release mold.

6. Snap on your drip shield.

7. Serve and Enjoy!

Nutritional Value - (Serving Size 1 Popsicle):

0 grams of Protein.

10 grams of Fat.

1 grams of Carbs.

104 Calories.

Keto Strawberry Cheesecake (Serves 8)

Ingredients:

Crust:

4 tablespoons of Butter

3/4 cup of Almond Flour

3/4 cup of Pecans

2 tablespoons of Splenda

Filling:

4 Eggs

9 Strawberries

1 1/2 pounds of Cream Cheese

1/2 tablespoon of Lemon Juice

1/2 tablespoon of Liquid Vanilla

1/4 cup of Sour Cream

1/2 teaspoon of EZ-Sweetz

Directions:

1. Preheat your oven to approximately 400 degrees.

2. Crush up your pecans.

3. In small saucepan, melt your butter and add in almond flour, pecans, and Splenda.

4. Mix crust in your saucepan for several minutes until your ingredients are combined.

5. Grease 9-inch springform pan. Line the bottom with your crust mixture.

6. Cook at 400 degrees approximately 7 minutes until your crust begins to brown.

7. Combine all filling ingredients in a stand mixer and combine well.

8. Slice some additional strawberries and line side of crust if you'd like.

9. Add your filling on top of your crust.

10. Top with more strawberries if you'd like.

11. Put cheesecake in your oven and drop it from 400 degrees to 250 degrees as soon as it's in the oven.

12. Cook approximately 60 to 90 minutes until your cheesecake has set.

13. Allow to cool.

14. Serve and Enjoy!

Nutritional Value - (Serving Size 1/8):

13 grams of Protein.

49 grams of Fat.

9 grams of Carbs.

535 Calories.

Keto Chocolate Cheesecake (Serves 8)

Ingredients:

Chocolate Crust

4 tablespoons of Butter

1 cup of Almond Flour

1/2 teaspoon of Cinnamon

1 tablespoon of Cocoa Powder

1 pinch of Salt

1/16 teaspoon of Stevia

Cheesecake Filling

2 Eggs

3/4 cup of Erythritol

16 ounces of Softened Cream Cheese

1/2 cup of Sour Cream

1 tablespoon of Cocoa Powder

1 teaspoon of Vanilla Extract

3 ounces of Unsweetened Baker's Chocolate

1 pinch of Salt

Directions:

1. Preheat your oven to 350 degrees.

2. Melt butter and combine with cinnamon, almond flour, Stevia, and cocoa powder. Mix together well.

3. Press this crust dough mixture into 9-inch springform pan and bake approximately 15 minutes till crust becomes solid and gets darker.

4. Begin making the cream cheese filling while crust bakes. Beat your erythritol and cream cheese with an electric hand mixer until it is smooth.

5. Add in vanilla extract, sour cream, eggs, and salt. Beat with mixer until it gets creamy.

6. Melt baker's chocolate in a small pan over low heat. Stir it constantly.

7. Pour chocolate and cocoa powder into your cream cheese mixture. Stir with your spatula to combine two mixtures.

8. Pour cheesecake batter into your pan on top of the crust.

9. Bake approximately 50 to 60 minutes until your cheesecake sets.

10. Allow to cool. I like to refrigerate it overnight.

11. Run knife around the edges of your pan to loosen cake.

12. Serve and Enjoy!

Nutritional Value - (Serving Size 1/8):

11.3 grams of Protein.

40 grams of Fat.

7.5 grams of Carbs.

450 Calories.

Red Velvet Cinnamon Cheesecakes (Serves 4)

Ingredients:

Red Velvet Layer

1 Egg

1/4 cup of Butter

1 tablespoon of Cocoa Powder

1 teaspoon of Red Food Coloring

1/2 teaspoon of Apple Cider Vinegar

1/2 teaspoon of Vanilla Extract

6 tablespoons of Almond Flour

Pinch of Salt

Cheesecake Layer

1 Egg

6 ounces of Cream Cheese

2 tablespoons of Erythritol

1 tablespoon of Butter

1/2 teaspoon of Vanilla Extract

1 teaspoon of Cinnamon

Pinch of Salt

Directions:

Red Velvet Layer

1. Preheat your oven to 350 degrees.

2. Melt butter in your small saucepan. Combine it with the erythritol. Keep the flame on low heat until your erythritol is dissolved.

3. In your mixing bowl, combine butter and erythritol with salt, vanilla, and cocoa powder.

4. Add in your egg and mix together until it is well combined.

5. Add in food coloring and your apple cider vinegar.

6. Add sifted almond flour and mix it together until fully combined.

7. Evenly pour your mixture among 4 greased ramekins. Be sure to tap a hard surface to flatten your batter out and remove the air bubbles. Place them on your cookie sheet and place them into your refrigerator while you're making your cheesecake layer.

Cheesecake Layer

1. Using your electric hand mixer, beat your softened cream cheese and butter until light and fluffy.

2. Add in vanilla extract, cinnamon, and egg. Beat your mixture again.

3. Add your powdered erythritol and salt. Mix with your electric hand mixer.

Combining

1. Take your ramekins out of refrigerator and spoon about 2 big teaspoons onto each of the red velvet layers. They shouldn't mix, but should meet without having any gaps between each of them.

2. Use your spoon to push the cheesecake layer to edges of your ramekins. Make sure there are no gaps between your ramekins and your cakes. Tap your ramekins again on a hard surface so your top layer will flatten out.

3. Bake in your oven for approximately 20 minutes. Make sure tops are set before removing from oven.

4. Allow to cool.

5. Serve and Enjoy!

Nutritional Value - (Serving Size 1/4):

17 grams of Protein.

36 grams of Fat.

2 grams of Carbs.

420 Calories.

Mini Cheesecakes (Serves 8)

Ingredients:

Cheesecake

1 Egg

8 ounces of Cream Cheese

1/4 cup of Erythritol

1/2 teaspoon of Lemon Juice

1/2 teaspoon of Vanilla Extract

Pinch of Salt

Crust

2 tablespoons of Butter

1/2 cup of Almond Meal

Directions:

1. Preheat your oven to 350 degrees.

2. To make your crust, melt butter until it is liquid and then mix with your almond meal.

3. Tale a teaspoon of dough at a time and press into bottom of your muffin tin. You can line your pan with cupcake liners to make removal easy.

4. Bake your crusts approximately 5 minutes at 350 degrees. Should be crispy and slightly brown.

5. Beat cream cheese with your electric hand mixer until it is creamy. Add in lemon, vanilla extract, erythritol, and egg. Beat until well combined.

6. Fill all the crust bottomed muffin tin cups. Do so evenly and nearly to the top.

7. Bake approximately 15 minutes at 350 degrees. Cheesecakes should be a little jiggly.

8. Allow to cool. I let them cool overnight.

9. Slide knife around outer edges of each cup to loosen.

10. Serve and Enjoy!

<u>Nutritional Value - (Serving Size 1 Mini Cheesecake):</u>

4 grams of Protein.

16 grams of Fat.

2 grams of Carbs.

176 Calories.

No Bake Lemon Cheesecake

Ingredients:

2 ounces of Heavy Cream

8 ounces of Softened Cream Cheese

1 tablespoon of Lemon Juice

1 teaspoon of Stevia Glycerite

1 teaspoon of Splenda

1 teaspoon of Vanilla Flavoring

Directions:

1. Mix all your ingredients together and then whip it into a pudding-like consistency. Spoon mixture into small serving cups and then refrigerate till it sets.

2. Serve and Enjoy!

White Chocolate Raspberry Cheesecake Fluff

Ingredients:

2 ounces of Heavy Cream

8 ounces of Softened Cream Cheese

1 teaspoon of Stevia Glycerite

1 tablespoon of Da Vinci Sugar-Free White Chocolate Flavor Syrup

1 teaspoon of Low Sugar Raspberry Preserves

Directions:

1. Mix all your ingredients together and then whip it into a pudding-like consistency. Spoon mixture into small serving cups and then refrigerate till it sets.

2. Serve and Enjoy!

Chocolate Chip Cheesecake

Ingredients:

2 ounces of Heavy Cream

8 ounces of Softened Cream Cheese

1 ounce of Mini Chocolate Chips

1 teaspoon of Splenda

1 teaspoon of Stevia Glycerite

Directions:

1. Mix all your ingredients together and then whip it into a pudding-like consistency. Spoon mixture into small serving cups and then refrigerate till it sets.

2. Serve and Enjoy!

Chocolate Cherry Cheesecake

Ingredients:

2 ounces of Heavy Cream

8 ounces of Softened Cream Cheese

1 teaspoon of Stevia Glycerite

1 tablespoon of Da Vince Sugar-Free Cherry Flavored Syrup

1 tablespoon of Dutch Process Cocoa Powder

3 to 5 drops of EZ-Sweet Liquid

Directions:

1. Mix all your ingredients together except EZ-Sweet and then whip it into a pudding-like consistency.

2. Add your EZ-Sweet a drop at a time to your mixture until it is sweet. Spoon mixture into small serving cups and then refrigerate until it sets.

3. Serve and Enjoy!

Chocolate Peanut Butter Truffles

Ingredients:

4 tablespoons of Melted Butter

1 cup of Peanut Butter

1.5 cups of Powdered Erythritol

6 ounces of Sugar-Free Chocolate (either chips or a bar)

Directions:

1. Melt butter.

2. Mix peanut butter, powdered erythritol, and melted butter together.

3. Scoop out 2 tablespoons of mixture and roll out into small balls. Lay on a baking sheet lined with parchment paper. Chill in your refrigerator for approximately 30 minutes.

4. Melt your chocolate in a small bowl for 10 to 20 seconds in your microwave. Stir it well.

5. Place one of your truffles in your bowl at a time and rotate it with a spoon so that chocolate covers every side. Take out and allow excess chocolate to fall off.

6. Place back on your baking sheet lined with parchment paper and place in refrigerator for another hour to chill.

7. Serve and Enjoy!

Nutritional Value - (Serving Size 1 Truffle):

5.9 grams of Protein.

17 grams of Fat.

5 grams of Carbs.

200 Calories.

Double Chocolate Bundt Cake (Serves 8)

Ingredients:

Bundt Cake

3 large Eggs

1 cup of Butter

2 cups of Anthony's Almond Flour

2 tablespoons of Coconut Flour

1 1/2 teaspoons of Baking Soda

1 cup of Erythritol

1/2 teaspoon of Salt

1 cup of Water

1/2 cup of Cocoa Powder

1/2 cup of Sour Cream

2 teaspoons of Vanilla Extract

White Chocolate Glaze

2 tablespoons of Heavy Cream

2 ounces of Anthony's Organic Cocoa Butter Wafers

1 teaspoon of Vanilla Extract

3 tablespoons of Powdered Erythritol

Topping

20 grams of Anthony's Organic Cocoa Nibs

Directions:

1. Preheat oven to 350 degrees.

2. Whisk together 2 cups of Anthony's Blanched Almond Flour with your baking soda, salt, coconut flour, and erythritol.

3. Heat up butter, water, and cocoa powder in a small pot over medium heat. Whisk until it is combined and then take off heat.

4. Pour half the chocolate mixture into your dry mix and stir it to combine. Once it thickens, pour in other half and stir to combine again.

5. Add 1 egg at a time to your mixture.

6. Add vanilla extract and sour cream. Stir well.

7. Pour your mixture into a greased bundt cake pan. Bake approximately 40 to 50 minutes.

8. Prepare glaze while cake bakes. Melt your cocoa butter wafers.

9. Add powdered erythritol and stir to combine. Add heavy cream and place in refrigerator. Take out and stir approximately every 5 minutes.

10. Once opaque and thick, pulse it using your Nutribullet or blend in blender until it is smooth.

11. Once cake is done baking, allow to cool in its pan for approximately 10 minutes. Invert onto a cooling rack on your baking sheet or plate. Allow to completely cool.

12. Glaze your cake. While glaze is wet, sprinkle your cocoa nibs over your cake. Let glaze cool down and harden.

13. Serve and Enjoy!

Nutritional Value - (Serving Size 1/8):

10 grams of Protein.

50 grams of Fat.

5 grams of Carbs.

520 Calories.

Chocolate Caramel Lave Cake (Serves 4)

Ingredients:

1/2 cup of Cocoa Powder

1/4 cup of Carolyn's Low-Carb Caramel Sauce

1/8 teaspoon of Powdered Stevia

1/4 cup of Erythritol

1/4 teaspoon of Salt

1/2 teaspoon of Cinnamon

1/4 cup of Melted Butter

1 teaspoon of Vanilla Extract

4 medium Eggs

Directions:

1. Prepare caramel sauce and allow to cool. Put some in a small jar and allow to freeze.

2. Preheat your oven to 350 degrees.

3. Prepare lava cake batter. Combine all your dry ingredients and mix to get out lumps.

4. Combine wet ingredients and mix with dry ingredients.

5. Spray 4 ramekins with oil or use some butter to grease them.

6. Fill ramekins halfway each with your batter.

7. Place tablespoon of caramel sauce into center of each of your ramekin, letting it rest on your lava cake batter.

8. Pour rest of your batter over caramel. Cover it completely.

9. Place your ramekins on baking sheet and bake approximately 13 minutes. Tops of cake should be set but still jiggle.

10. Allow to relax approximately 3 minutes. Run sharp knife around edges of the ramekin to loosen your cakes.

11. Place your plate upside down onto your ramekin. Flip ramekin and plate so ramekin is now facing upside down on your plate. Tap ramekin to make your cake gently fall onto your plate.

12. Add your desired optional toppings. I like whip cream and berries.

13. Serve and Enjoy.

Nutritional Value - (Serving Size 1 Cake):

8 grams of Protein.

24 grams of Fat.

6 grams of Carbs.

230 Calories.

Keto Lava Cake (Serves 1)

Ingredients:

1 medium Egg

2 tablespoons of Erythritol

2 tablespoons of Cocoa Powder

1/2 teaspoon of Vanilla Extract

1 tablespoon of Heavy Cream

1/4 teaspoon of Baking Powder

Pinch of Salt

Directions:

1. Preheat your oven to 350 degrees.

2. Combine cocoa powder and erythritol. Mix until it is smooth. Remove any clumps that form.

3. In a separate bowl, beat egg till fluffy.

4. Add heavy cream, vanilla extract, and egg to your cocoa mixture. Add in baking soda and salt.

5. Spray cooking oil into your mug and pour your batter in. Bake for approximately 10 to 15 minutes at 350 degrees. The top should be set but still jiggly.

6. Allow to relax approximately 3 minutes. Run sharp knife around edges of the ramekin to loosen your cakes.

7. Place your plate upside down onto your mug. Flip mug and plate so mug is now facing upside down on your plate. Tap mug to make your cake gently fall onto your plate.

8. Add your desired optional toppings. I like to add a scoop of ice cream on top.

9. Serve and Enjoy.

Nutritional Value:

8 grams of Protein.

13 grams of Fat.

4 grams of Carbs.

173 Calories.

Pink Lemonade Cloud Cake (Serves 2)

Ingredients:

Layers:

1 Oopsie Roll

1/4 teaspoon of Powdered Stevia

Frosting:

2 tablespoons of Erythritol

1/3 cup of Softened Butter

1 teaspoon of Fresh Lemon Juice

1 teaspoon of Lemon Zest

2 Strawberries

1 tablespoon of Heavy Cream

1/2 teaspoon of Poppy Seeds

Pinch of Salt

Directions:

1. Make your oopsie rolls. If you want them to be sweeter add some Stevia to your batter while making them.

2. Once cooked and you've allowed to cool, use a mug to stamp out uniformly sized circles of your oopsie rolls.

3. Once the layers are ready, beat your erythritol and butter until it is creamy. Add a tablespoon of your cream, lemon zest, and lemon juice.

4. Add poppy seeds and finely chopped strawberries.

5. Place frosting mixture into Ziploc bag and remove as much air as possible before twisting the bag and snipping the top.

6. Lay an oopsie roll on your plate and frost the outside of the cake. Follow up by filling in the middle.

7. Stack another oopsie roll on top of the frosted oopsie roll and gently press down. Repeat the previous step. Do this until you have 3 layers of oopsie rolls.

8. Garnish with frosting and your walnut.

9. Chill in refrigerator for approximately 1 hour.

10. Serve and Enjoy!

Nutritional Value - (Serving Size 1/2):

6.5 grams of Protein.

42 grams of Fat.

3 grams of Carbs.

430 Calories.

Flourless Chocolate Cake (Serves 8)

Ingredients:

3 Eggs

4 ounces of Unsweetened Baker's Chocolate

1/2 cup of Cocoa Powder

1/2 cup of Butter

1 teaspoon of Vanilla Extract

1 cup of Swerve Erythritol (separated into 1/2 cup, 1/4 cup, 1/4 cup)

1/2 teaspoon of Salt

Directions:

1. Preheat oven to 300 degrees. Set up your double boiler to melt your butter and baker's chocolate together. If no boiler use your pan over low heat.

2. Once they are both melted, combine them both together. Add in 1/2 cup of erythritol and stir well over low flame until it is dissolved.

3. Separate 3 eggs and beat eggs whites until they get foamy. Add 1/4 cup of erythritol slowly while beating egg whites. Should form stiff peaks and turn glossy.

4. Clean beaters and beat your 3 egg yolks. Slowly add in last 1/4 cup of erythritol. Yolks should turn pale yellow and double in volume.

5. Add in chocolate mixture to egg yolks. Stir well.

6. Add in cocoa powder. Stir well. Add salt and vanilla.

7. Add a third of your egg whites and fold in gently. Repeat process until all the eggs whites have been added and folded in.

8. Spray your springform pan with some cooking oil. Pour in your chocolate batter. Bake approximately 35 minutes.

9. Dust with some powdered erythritol.

10. Serve and Enjoy!

Nutritional Value - (Serving Size 1/8):

5.6 grams of Protein.

21 grams of Fat.

2 grams of Carbs.

240 Calories.

Chocolate Covered Strawberries

Ingredients:

1/2 pound of Fresh Strawberries

1 tablespoon of Coconut Oil

2 ounces of Chocolate Chips

2 tablespoons of Coconut Butter

Directions:

1. Melt chocolate chips. Stir well.

2. Remove from any heat and add in coconut oil and coconut butter until everything is melted. Move to a small bowl.

3. Dry strawberries. Grab by stem and dip into the chocolate.

4. Place chocolate strawberries on baking sheet lined with parchment paper and refrigerate for approximately 1 hour.

5. Serve and Enjoy!

Raspberry Cream Crepes

Ingredients:

Crepes:

2 Eggs

2 ounces of Cream Cheese

2 tablespoons of Erythritol

Dash of Cinnamon

Pinch of Salt

Filling

3 ounces of Raspberries

1/2 cup + 2 tablespoons of Whole Milk Ricotta

Toppings:

Sugar-Free Maple Syrup

Whipped Cream

Directions:

1. Combine all crepe ingredients into food processor or blender. Blend together for approximately 20 seconds so no chunks remain.

2. Heat your pan over medium heat. Spray with your cooking spray and put a 1/4 of your batter at a time. While pouring, tilt pan onto all sides so your crepe batter reaches each edge of the pan.

3. Let your crepe cook for approximately 1 minute. Then wedge your spatula underneath and wiggle gently until you reach the center and flip it. Let cook another 15 seconds.

4. Continue doing this process until all your batter is gone. Should make 5 or 6 crepes in total.

5. Let crepes cool. Lay next to one another not on top of each other.

6. Stuff them with your whole ricotta cheese.

7. Add your raspberries.

8. Fold each side of crepe over your filling and press down gently to seal it.

9. Add toppings.

10. Serve and Enjoy!

<u>Nutritional Value:</u>

15 grams of Protein.

40 grams of Fat.

8 grams of Carbs.

570 Calories.

Pumpkin Pecan Tart (Serves 2)

Ingredients:

Crust

1 teaspoon of Cinnamon

1/2 cup of Almond Flour

2 tablespoons of Melted Butter

Pinch of Salt

Filling

1/2 cup of Pumpkin Puree

1/2 cup of Ricotta Cheese

1 teaspoon of Cinnamon

1/4 teaspoon of Pumpkin Pie Spice

2 tablespoons of Erythritol

1/2 teaspoon of Vanilla Extract

1 Egg

1 Egg White

Pinch of Salt

Topping

Sugar-Free Maple Syrup

16 Pecans

Directions:

1. Preheat your oven to 350 degrees. Combine crust ingredients in a bowl.

2. Mix well and press into your mini tartlet pans. I used 4 1/2 inch pans. Let your tart crusts bake in oven approximately 10 minutes. Let cool while you work on the filling.

3. Combine egg, egg white, pumpkin puree, and ricotta cheese.

4. Mix in the rest of the filling ingredients. Stir well to combine.

5. Once crusts are cooled, pour your filling onto your crusts. Place tart pans on baking sheet and bake approximately 20 minutes.

6. Remove from oven and add pecans to top. Place back in your oven approximately 10 minutes. The tops should have set yet still be jiggly.

7. Let cool. Drizzle maple syrup on top.

8. Serve and Enjoy!

Nutritional Value - (Serving Size 1/2):

19 grams of Protein.

45 grams of Fat.

9 grams of Carbs.

530 Calories.

Sugar-Free Panna Cotta (Serves 4)

Ingredients:

1 cup of Unsweetened Almond Milk

1 cup of Heavy Cream

1/3 cup of Erythritol

1 sachet of Unflavored Gelatin

1 tablespoon of Fresh Lemon Juice

1 teaspoon of Vanilla Extract

1/2 cup of Sugar-Free Raspberry Jam

Raspberries

Directions:

1. In your saucepan, combine the almond milk and heavy cream over a low flame.

2. Add your gelatin and erythritol. Allow to dissolve in your warm cream. Don't allow to boil.

3. Use your whisk to stir it together well.

4. Turn off heat and add your lemon juice and vanilla extract.

5. Grease 4 cups or ramekins. Spray with oil and pour your batter into each one evenly.

6. Cover your cup or ramekin with plastic wrap and place in refrigerator for a minimum of 2 hours.

7. Take out and run a knife around edges. Flip over onto a plate.

8. Top with your raspberry jam and fresh raspberries.

9. Serve and Enjoy!

Nutritional Value - (Serving Size 1/4):

1 gram of Protein.

12 grams of Fat.

11 grams of Carbs.

131 Calories.

Pumpkin Maple Flaxseed Muffins (Serves 10)

Ingredients:

1 Egg

1/3 cup of Erythritol

1/2 tablespoon of Baking Powder

1 1/4 cups of Ground Flaxseeds

1 tablespoon of Cinnamon

1 cup of Pure Pumpkin Puree

1/2 teaspoon of Salt

1 tablespoon of Pumpkin Pie Spice

1/4 cup of Walden Farm's Maple Syrup

2 tablespoons of Coconut Oil

1/2 teaspoon of Vanilla Extract

1/2 teaspoon of Apple Cider Vinegar

Directions:

1. Add some cupcake liners to your muffin tin. Preheat oven to 350 degrees.

2. Grind flaxseeds for 1 second in your Nutribullet.

3. Combine your dry ingredients and stir well to disperse evenly.

4. Add your pumpkin puree. Mix well.

5. Add you vanilla extract, maple syrup, and pumpkin spice.

6. Add in your coconut oil, apple cider vinegar mix, and egg. Mix well.

7. Add a large tablespoon of mixture to each muffin liner and top with pumpkin seeds. Allow some room for muffins to rise.

8. Bake approximately 20 minutes. Tops should brown slightly.

9. Allow to cool. Add any toppings or butter to muffins.

10. Serve and Enjoy.

Nutritional Value - (Serving Size 1 Muffin):

4.7 grams of Protein.

8.4 grams of Fat.

2.2 grams of Carbs.

120 Calories.

Pumpkin Spice Creme Brulee (Serves 2)

Ingredients:

2 Egg Yolks

1 cup of Heavy Cream

2 tablespoons of Erythritol

1 teaspoon of Pumpkin Pie Spice

2 tablespoons of Pumpkin Puree

Directions:

1. Preheat your oven to 300 degrees. Heat heavy cream in saucepan. Don't allow to boil. Add in pumpkin pie spice once your cream begins to bubble. Turn off the heat and cover with your lid. Allow to stand for 5 minutes.

2. Separate two egg yolks and then whisk until they're both light yellow.

3. Add some of your cream mixture at a time to your eggs while continuously whisking.

4. Once combined, add your pumpkin puree. Whisk together well.

5. Add in erythritol. Mix well.

6. Place 2 ramekins in your deep baking dish and fill with hot water (approximately 1/2 way up ramekins).

7. Pour mixture into ramekins and bake approximately 30 to 40 minutes. Tops of creme brulees will be set but jiggly.

8. Allow to cool approximately 15 minutes. Place in refrigerator at least 4 hours.

9. Sprinkle some erythritol on top if you desire extra sweetness.

10. Use a blowtorch to burn tops of your creme brulees. Can also place in broiler for 1 to 2 minutes if you don't have a torch.

11. Serve and Enjoy!

Nutritional Value - (Serving Size):

5 grams of Protein.

49 grams of Fat.

5 grams of Carbs.

460 Calories.

Salted Caramel Panna Cotta (Serves 4)

Ingredients:

1/4 cup of Erythritol

2 cups of Heavy Cream

1 teaspoon of Vanilla

1 sachet of Unflavored Gelatin

1/2 cup of Caramel

Directions:

1. Heat up cream in a saucepan over low heat. Add in erythritol and gelatin. Don't allow to boil or simmer.

2. Use your whisk to stir together well. Add in your vanilla extract and stir well.

3. Grease your ramekins and wipe excess with a paper towel.

4. Pour your mixture into ramekins and chill at least 2 hours.

5. Pour 2 tablespoons of caramel over each ramekin of panna cotta.

6. Serve and Enjoy!

Nutritional Value - (Serving Size 1/4):

2 grams of Protein.

44 grams of Fat.

6 grams of Carbs.

450 Calories.

Keto Truffles (Serves 12)

Ingredients:

2 tablespoons of Honey

150 grams of Organic Dark Chocolate

1/2 cup of Organic Heavy Cream

2 tablespoons of Grass Fed Butter

2 tablespoons of Raw Cocoa Powder

1/2 teaspoon of Cinnamon

1/2 teaspoon of Pure Vanilla Extract

Pinch of Sea Salt

Directions:

1. Heat cream over the low flame. Don't allow to boil.

2. Chop chocolate into small pieces.

3. When simmering add in your chocolate and stir until it is combined with cream. Add in your butter and stir in until it is melted completely.

4. Turn off heat and add your cinnamon, vanilla, honey, and salt. Mix well to combine.

5. Place in refrigerator for approximately 1 hour. Stir every 20 minutes.

6. Once cooled and hardened, scoop some of your mixture out and roll into small balls about 1 1/2 inches in diameter.

7. Place each truffle ball on a baking sheet lined with parchment paper and refrigerate approximately 30 minutes.

8. Roll in hands to smooth balls out. Place your cocoa powder in a bowl and add your truffles. Shake and roll them in your cocoa powder to coat evenly.

9. Serve and Enjoy!

Nutritional Value - (Serving Size 1 Truffle):

1.3 grams of Protein.

12 grams of Fat.

5.6 grams of Carbs.

142 Calories.

Strawberry Pistachio Creamsicle (Serves 4)

Ingredients:

8 ounces of Strawberries

1/2 cup of Heavy Cream

2 ounces of Salted Pistachios

1/2 cup of Almond Milk

2 doonk scoops of Stevia

Directions:

1. Place popsicle molds in the freezer beforehand to accelerate freezing process.

2. Blend your heavy cream, strawberries, almond milk, and Stevia until it is fully combined. Blend for a minute.

3. Throw in pistachios and stir. Do not blend.

4. Pour your creamsicle mix into the cold popsicle molds and insert your bases. Freeze approximately 2 hours until it has set.

5. Remove creamsicles by running hot water on the outside of molds. Gently pull out.

6. Serve and Enjoy!

Nutritional Value - (Serving Size 1 Creamsicle):

4 grams of Protein.

12.5 grams of Fat.

5.g grams of Carbs.

158 Calories.

Keto Caramel (Serves 4)

Ingredients:

4 tablespoons of Heavy Cream

4 tablespoons of Unsalted Butter

1 teaspoon of Erythritol

Pinch of Salt

Directions:

1. Melt your butter in pan and cook until it is golden brown.

2. Pour in heavy cream and combine. Lower your heat and simmer approximately 1 minute.

3. Add in erythritol. Allow to dissolve and add your salt.

4. Cook until it gets stickier and thicker.

5. Pour into glass container and continue to stir caramel mixture while it cools down and thickens.

Nutritional Value - (Serving Size 1/4):

0 grams of Protein.

17 grams of Fat.

0.5 grams of Carbs.

163 Calories.

Keto Skillet Brownies (Serves 4)

Ingredients:

Brownies

1 Egg

6 tablespoons of Butter

1/3 cup of Cocoa Powder

1/3 cup of Erythritol

1/2 teaspoon of Vanilla Extract

1/4 cup of Almond Flour

1/4 cup of Walnuts

1/2 teaspoon of Baking Powder

Pinch of Salt

Peanut Butter Drizzle

1 tablespoon of Butter

1 tablespoon of Peanut butter

Directions:

1. Preheat your oven to 350 degrees.

2. Melt butter in small pan and add in erythritol. Allow to dissolve.

3. Pour mixture into mixing bowl and add in salt, vanilla extract, and cocoa powder.

4. Add in your egg and beat until it is well combined.

5. Add your baking powder and almond flour.

6. Fold in your choice of nuts. I used walnuts.

7. Pour brownie batter into your 6-inch cast iron skillet.

8. Place in oven and bake approximately 30 minutes. The top will be set but still jiggly.

9. Add peanut butter drizzle if you desire.

10. Serve and Enjoy!

Nutritional Value - (Serving Size 1/4):

5.8 grams of Protein.

31.3 grams of Fat.

3 grams of Carbs.

333 Calories.

Keto Apple Pie (Serves 8)

Ingredients:

Crust

4 Eggs

1 cup of Grass Fed Butter

1 1/2 cups of Coconut Flour

1/2 teaspoon of Salt

Filling

1/4 cup of Honey

6 Macintosh Apples

1 teaspoon of Vanilla Extract

1 tablespoon of Cinnamon

2 tablespoons of Grass Fed Butter

Directions:

1. Preheat oven to 425 degrees.

2. Melt 1 cup of grass fed butter and combine with eggs and whisk it together.

3. Add salt and coconut flour.

4. Divide mixture in half and roll one of your halves into a ball and press and flatten it to your greased 9-inch pie pan.

5. With your other 1/2 of dough, roll and flatten into 1/4 inch of thickness. Place to the side.

6. Peel and slice your apples into desired size pieces.

7. Toss apple pieces, vanilla extract, honey, and cinnamon into a bowl. Make sure apples are all evenly coated in your mixture.

8. Pour your apples into crust lined pan. Place butter on top to allow it to brown and moisten your filling. Cover piece with your rolled out dough that you put to the side. Seal all the edges by pinching them. Slice a few slits on top of your dough so some steam can come out in the oven when cooking.

9. Separate an egg. Whisk the white part. Use a kitchen brush to brush some of the egg on the entire top crust.

10. Place in oven and bake approximately 15 minutes at 425 degrees. Lower to 350 degrees and continue baking another 40 minutes.

11. Let cool slightly until it is warm.

Nutritional Value - (Serving Size 1/8):

8 grams of Protein.

32 grams of Fat.

27 grams of Carbs.

450 Calories.

Gluten Free Banana Bread (Serves 8)

Ingredients:

Wet Ingredients

1 Juiced Orange

3 Ripe Bananas

Pinch of Orange Zest

1/4 cup of Honey

2 tablespoons of Coconut Oil

1/4 teaspoon of Vanilla Extract

Dry Ingredients

3/4 teaspoon of Cinnamon

1/2 teaspoon of Salt

1 1/3 cup of Almond Flour

1/8 teaspoon of Cayenne

1 teaspoon of Baking Powder

1/2 teaspoon of Baking Soda

1 teaspoon of Xanthan Gum

Fold-Ins

3/4 cups of Flaxseeds

2 Grated Carrots

1/4 teaspoon of Grated Fresh Ginger

3/4 cup of Chopped Walnuts

Topping

Coconut Butter

Honey

Directions:

1. Preheat your oven to 410 degrees.

2. Mash bananas until a thick wet mush.

3. Add orange zest and juiced orange.

4. Add in vanilla extract, honey, and coconut oil.

5. Add in all dry ingredients.

6. Shred ginger and carrots. Fold into mixture. Roughly chop walnuts. Throw into your mixture.

7. Fold in rest of ingredients.

8. Grease your medium sized bread pan with some butter or coconut oil. Pour in your batter. Feel free to sprinkle on sugar or drizzle some honey at the end.

9. Bake approximately 25 minutes at 410 degrees. Lower temperature to 350 degrees and bake approximately 30 minutes.

10. Allow to cool and then slice bread.

11. Serve and Enjoy!

Nutritional Value - (Serving Size 1/8):

8 grams of Protein.

24 grams of Fat.

23 grams of Carbs.

357 Calories.

Homemade Chocolate Chips (Serves 3)

Ingredients:

1 Low-Carb Chocolate Bar

Directions:

1. Melt your chocolate bar.

2 Pour chocolate onto silicone pot holder.

3. Place in freezer and allow to freeze approximately 2 hours.

4. When frozen, twist your silicone molds and pop out your chips onto a small plate.

5. Serve and Enjoy!

Nutritional Value - (Serving Size 1/3):

0.2 grams of Protein.

2.8 grams of Fat.

0.1 grams of Carbs.

27.5 Calories.

Homemade Nutella (Serves 12)

Ingredients:

2 cups of Hazelnuts

1 tablespoon of Coconut Oil

1/4 cup of Cocoa Powder

1/4 cup of Heavy Cream

1 teaspoon of Vanilla Extract

1/4 cup of Water

1/4 teaspoon of Salt

1/2 cup of Erythritol

Directions:

1. Preheat oven to 325 degrees.

2. Spread cookie sheet and spread hazelnuts evenly on one layer. Roast approximately 10 to 15 minutes.

3. Allow nuts to cool. Put nuts in a towel and rub them vigorously.

4. Once nuts have skins off, drop them into your food processor. Blend for a few minutes until it looks like peanut butter.

5. If sticking to sides add a little coconut oil and scrape down the sides.

6. Add in rest of ingredients. Continue to blend and scrape the sides.

7. Remove from blender once thoroughly mixed and place in a container.

8. Serve and Enjoy!

Nutritional Value - (Serving Size 1/12):

3 grams of Protein.

15 grams of Fat.

2 grams of Carbs.

162 Calories.

Nutella Sundae (Serves 2)

Ingredients:

4 scoops of Low-Carb Ice Cream

2 Strawberries

2 tablespoons of Homemade Nutella

Whipped Cream

Sprinkles

Directions:

1. Mix it all together.

2. Place in a bowl.

3. Add your toppings.

4. Serve and Enjoy!

Nutritional Value - (Serving Size 1/2):

4 grams of Protein.

14 grams of Fat.

10 grams of Carbs.

191 Calories.

Nutella Brownies (Serves 4)

Ingredients:

4 Eggs

1 Cup of Nutella

4 tablespoons of Erythritol

Directions:

1. Preheat oven to 350 degrees.

2. Place Nutella in a microwave for approximately 15-second intervals, stirring until it gets really soft.

3. Crack eggs and mix with electric mixer until they've tripled in volume and become a lighter yellow color. Should take 5 to 8 minutes.

4. Combine Nutella and eggs. Whisk until it is combined. Add your erythritol.

5. Add mixture to ramekins. Put ramekins on cookie sheet. Bake approximately 25 to 30 minutes.

6. Let it cool.

7. Serve and Enjoy!

Nutritional Value - (Serving Size 1/4):

12 grams of Protein.

35 grams of Fat.

4 grams of Carbs.

396 Calories.

Conclusion

Thanks for reading my book. I hope this diet guide has provided you with all the information you needed to get going. Don't put off getting started. The sooner you begin the sooner you'll start to notice an improvement in your health and well-being. While results won't come overnight, they will come if you stick to the information found in this book.

I also hope you enjoy all the recipes I've included. There's no shortage of meals you can enjoy on a ketogenic diet. I've tried to include all the tools I use in my section on keto kitchen tools. This way you'll know exactly what I use to help aid me in making these healthy delicious meals. If you still have unanswered questions I suggest checking out one of the resource sites or apps I discussed. When I first got started out these sites had all the answers I needed. They were an invaluable resource to have at my disposal.

Good luck. I wish you nothing but the best!